KETO FOR WOMAN AFTER 50

The Ultimate Ketogenic Diet Step by
Step To Learn How to Easily Lose
Weight for Woman and Feel Younger

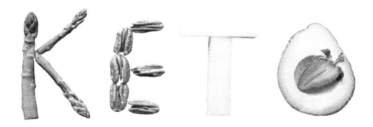

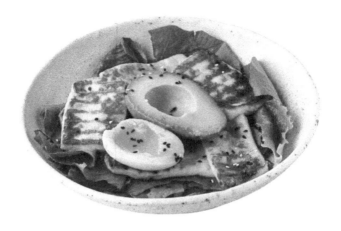

Table of Contents

Introduction

The increasing age, deterioration in physiological function, metabolic dysfunction, poor immunity makes a person vulnerable to a number of chronic diseases. So, you now have to start worrying about your health if you're over 50. Picture what life would be like, when a simple diet change could almost immediately make you look years younger.

The keto diet, particularly for weight loss, is very common worldwide because of its many advantages. You will just be capable of taking your body to a whole new level when you adopt this diet and regain the youthful nature also after 50 years of age.

Ketogenic diets and Atkins allow followers to eliminate carbohydrates from their foods. Thus, while the Atkins diet lowers the calories steadily over time, Keto sets strict limits on carbohydrates and protein. The carbohydrate system is depleted by this eating practice, forcing it to consume fat and help create an extra supply of energy called ketones. A conventional ketogenic diet restricts carbohydrates to less than 10% of calories and 20% of protein, while the rest is fat.

Losing weight is only the beginning. Research has demonstrated a stabilized emotional state. It enhances energy rates. Regulate your blood sugar. It lowers blood pressure, boosts potassium, and many have personally seen the outcomes in their lives.

In addition to traditional therapies, including chemotherapy for many other cancers that affect women, including glioblastoma multiforme, aggressive cancer that affects the brain, the ketogenic diet so far has shown potential results when used as a treatment.

Today, life is characterized by packaged and refined food containing tons of sugar, low energy, anxiety, and depression. Many people are frightened by Keto. They may not have a decent amount of money to eat these. Or perhaps they are afraid of losing their favorite meal.

The insights and recipes included in this guide can get you started on your journey to a healthy, fitter body, even though you suffer from age-related ailments or obesity over the age of 50 years.

Chapter 1: Keto Diet

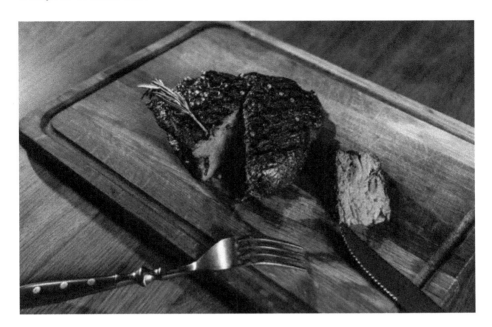

Looking to lose weight and keep in shape as you get on in years can be very challenging, especially when you're a woman. Your body is not as supple as it used to be once, and the body's metabolism has been slowed down to a great extent. But it doesn't need to be like that. There's a way to accelerate one's metabolism and be the healthiest and fittest version one has ever been, and you will get to know about that all in the Keto Diet.

1.1 How does body routine requirements modify once the 50-year Rubicon is reached?

You often come across people who have a high metabolism rate. Such people, despite consuming large quantities of food are slim. That quick metabolism very effectively processes that food. Now, these people do not only have a metabolism that is genetically fast, but they may also be younger and may also have more lean muscle mass, which will more effectively burn the calories. They may also be individuals who consume a lot of calories, but they will be balanced calories such as proteins, fats, or carbohydrates.

1.2 Simple comprehension of keto diet mechanism

The concept of weight loss in the ketogenic diet is that alternative fuel ketones are produced from the stored fat if one deprives the body of glucose (thus "keto" genic) — the essential energy source for all body cells obtained from eating fatty foods. The brain's routine requirement of glucose is about 120 g a day, most often in constant supply, so glucose could not really be processed in there. The body first eliminates the stored glucose from the liver by fasting, even though when too little carbohydrate is consumed, and breaks down the muscle momentarily to eliminate glucose. As this occurs for 3- 4 days before the stored glucose becomes completely depleted, hormone blood levels are named insulin to drop. The body begins using fat as a primary energy source. The liver makes ketone bodies out of fat, which can be used when there is no glucose available.

The term is called Ketosis, when the ketone bodies start to gather in one's body. When the ketone bodies start to gather in one's body, the term is called Ketosis. Normally, young individuals experience mild Ketosis through fasting periods (e.g., nighttime sleeping) and very rigorous training. Proponents of the ketogenic diet suggest that if the diet is followed very carefully, blood levels of ketones will not reach a harmful amount ('ketoacidosis') because the brain will use ketones for food, and healthy young people can produce adequate insulin to prevent the formation of excessive ketones. How rapidly Ketosis occurs and the number of ketone bodies circulating in the blood varies from person to person, based on factors such as body fat percentage and metabolic rest rate.

1.3 What are the relevant considerations for women over the age of 50

Over the increasing age, the metabolic rate starts to slow down. You appear to conserve more calories with age. The metabolic rate could also be modified by the food types you consume, how much you eat certain foods, and your physical activity level. If women over 50 years of age person don't really reduce their calorie intake as they tend to age, and their physical activity does not increase, they may begin to gain weight.

1.4 How to get yourself inspired for the Keto adopted lifestyle.

Temptation, desires, social stigma, physical exhaustion, and mental grogginess ("keto fog") may cause those uncertain of what lies ahead to suddenly quit and return to their former foods over the first few weeks.

During those inaugural weeks, when the body is totally shifting its primary energy source from carbs to fats, here are a few ways to stay on track.

1.   Regularly update the necessities

When adopting the keto lifestyle, choose to make sure you get all the nutrients you really need while your general health is in tip-top condition. Just because you shift to Keto, this doesn't really mean you're going to start eating awful stodgy items. Do not follow those websites that are boring. Keto could be fun-loving. This isn't about consuming trash. It's about offering only what your body needs, and that also includes your taste buds.

2.   Keto-friendly holiday feast with mates

What's worse than being that guy on the table in a restaurant who can't eat anything? Before heading out, prepare your homework. Check out the popular suggested restaurants to find out if there is anything on the menu that suits you. Browse the restaurants' online menus or pick up a telephone to reach them. It's fantastic to have a dream restaurant. Find it out and visit these for your pleasure with your mates and enjoy a perfect holiday keto feast.

3.   Staying hydrated while working out a bit more

Regular exercise helps remove the glycogen in one's system, helping you to more quickly burn the calories on Keto. It'll take a couple of days for your body to adapt to the Keto diet and begin to achieve the results you're looking for in weight loss. So, don't be hard on yourself. Slow and gradual workouts do the trick.

It's always necessary to remain hydrated when eating the right stuff. Get a refillable water bottle. Take it with you and fill it, striving for at least 2 liters of water a day. Keeping healthful with stress-free exercises, helps the body to pass through Ketosis and take away more fat while being beneficial for the whole body, soul, and mind.

4. Don't obsess & get ready to feel smart

You shouldn't really be worrying 24 hours a day about what next to eat on Keto. Yes, particularly at first, the diet seems intense, but it does not have to be the entire focus of your day. When you strike the sweet spot of energy, do this on work or hobbies and embrace it. It is believed that Ketosis shakes out brain fog. If that sounds right to you, this could be a perfect time to start a new project at work that needs intense focus.

5. Prepare yourself for compliments.

It's good and fun to say that you're on Keto and have lost weight, you're going to be praised by people in your life, and that's motivating. You can lose five pounds and then, for no reason at all, regain it. It's not you—it's a natural adaptation of your body. Shrug it off and continue to move on. Eating a wide range of healthy foods on Keto keeps your levels of nutrients high and avoids boredom to boot.

1.5 How to minimize common misconceptions

1. Nervous about eating too much fat

When people start Keto, they sometimes do not consume adequate fat because our culture has been conditioned to assume that fats can make you fat. Since you're reducing keto carb intake, it's important to replace those calories with fat calories. If you just don't have enough calories, your hormonal function and metabolism can be affected in the long term. All fats really aren't considered equal, and since fats are the basis of the ketogenic diet, it is important that the right sources of fat are eaten.

2. There Isn't enough Sodium Intake

When one's body runs on ketones for energy, sodium is released alongside the water. You may fall prey to the dreaded flu, which is the primary cause for not substituting your electrolytes if you do not switch your sodium on Keto. To stop this, boost sodium intake by salting each meal, introducing pink Himalayan sea salt to your water and drinking it during the day, and also consuming broth from bouillon cubes, boost your sodium intake.

3. Too much obsession with the scale

While the ketogenic diet is recognized for its immense weight loss benefits, an accurate reading is not always shown on the scale. You will experience water weight loss over the first few days after starting Keto for the first time. But it will hold some water until the body has adjusted to this new type of diet. Several times a day, testing your weight would just prevent you from holding on to the ketogenic diet because weights normally fluctuate.

1.6 Can this ketogenic diet pose any danger to women?

Interestingly, although some research suggests that some risk factors for heart disease, including LDL (bad) cholesterol, may be increased by the ketogenic diet, however other studies have shown that the diet may support heart health.

Whether you should follow the keto diet relies on many factors. It is important to weigh the positive and negative aspects of the diet, as well as its suitability, based on your current state of health before you begin any major dietary changes.

For instance, for a woman with obesity, diabetes, or who is unable to lose weight or control her blood sugar by using dietary changes, the ketogenic diet may be an acceptable alternative. On the other hand, the diet is not safe for pregnant or breastfeeding women.

While some women may find success in adopting a ketogenic dietary pattern, it is probably more effective for the majority of women to pursue a less restrictive, healthy diet that can be maintained for life

Rely on your health and nutritional requirements, and it's often recommended to follow a dietary pattern that is rich in whole, nutritionally sound foods that can be preserved for life

1.7 Certain benefits of Keto for fitness

Surveys have shown that diet can benefit a large range of different health conditions.

- Cancer: The diet is currently being considered as an alternative cancer treatment, as it could help delay the growth of tumors.

- Ovarian polycystic syndrome: Insulin levels may also be lowered by a ketogenic diet, which can play a vital role in polycystic ovary syndrome.

- Alzheimer's disease: The keto diet will help relieve Alzheimer's disease symptoms and delay its development.

- Brain injuries: Some findings indicate that this diet can improve the results of brain trauma injuries.

- Epilepsy: Current study has also shown that a ketogenic diet in epileptic children can cause substantial reductions in seizures.

Chapter 2: Breakfast Recipes

1. Classic bacon and eggs

Cook time: 10 mins, Servings: 4, Difficulty: easy

Ingredients

- Eggs 8
- Sliced bacon 9.oz
- Cherry tomatoes (optional)

- Thyme (Fresh)

Instructions

1. On medium heat, fry the bacon in a saucepan until it gets crispy. Hold it aside on a plate. The rendered fat is to be left in the pan.

2. The same pan is used for frying the eggs. Pan is placed over medium heat, and eggs are cracked into the bacon grease. To prevent splattering of hot grease, you can also break them into a measuring cup and then carefully pour them into the pan.

3. Cook the eggs the way you prefer them. Let the eggs fry on one side for a sunny side up and cover the pan with a lid to ensure they are fried on top. Continue cooking for another 1 minute and then flip the eggs. Cherry tomatoes are cut in half and simultaneously fried.

4. Add pepper and salt to taste.

Nutrition

Kcal: 377, fat 32 g, Protein 20 g, net carbs one g.

2. Spinach and feta breakfast scramble

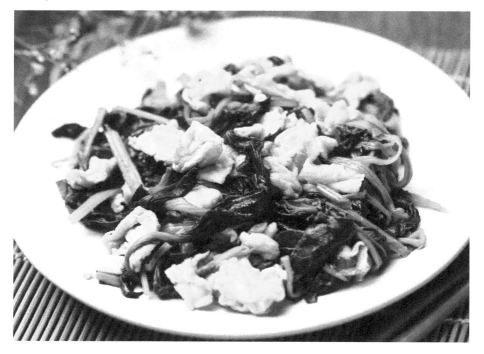

Cook time: 5-10 mins, Servings: 2, Difficulty: easy

Ingredients

- Large eggs 4
- Whipping cream2 tbsp. (heavy)
- Butter 2 tbsps.
- Baby spinach fresh 4 oz.
- Clove of garlic (minced)1
- Black pepper (salt and ground)
- Crumbled feta cheese 1½ oz. Feta
- Bacon 4 oz.

Instructions

1. We whisk the eggs and cream together in a medium bowl until well blended.

2. Over medium-low heat, the large skillet is heated, and then butter is added. Stir the spinach and garlic and let the butter melt. Cook till the spinach is wilted. Use salt and pepper to sprinkle.

3. The egg mixture is poured into the skillet and cooked until it starts to set around the edges. Gently lift the batter with the help of a rubber spatula from the edge of the pan towards the center. Continue to turn and lift until the eggs are set according to your taste.

4. Take off the pan from the stove and sprinkle feta cheese. Add a few fried bacon slices depending on your liking and serve quickly.

Nutrition

Kcal: 348, fat 30 g, Protein 16 g, net carbs 3 g

3. Dairy-free keto latte

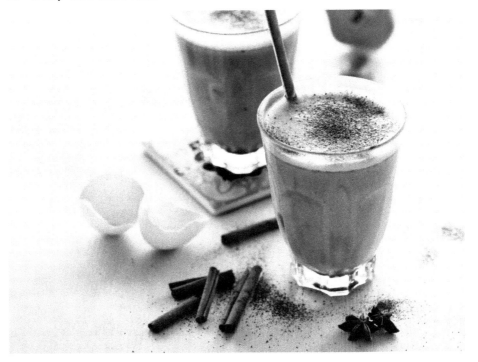

Cook time: 5 mins, Servings: 2, Difficulty: easy

Ingredients

- Eggs 2
- Coconut oil 2 tbsps.
- Cups of coffee 1 1/2
- Extract of vanilla1 pinch
- Pumpkin pie spice(ground ginger) 1 tsp

Instructions

1. Blend in a blender with all the ingredients. You have to be quick so that the eggs do not cook in the boiling water. Immediately drink.

Nutrition

Kcal 193, fat 18 g, Protein 6 g, net carbs 1 g

4. Avocado eggs served with bacon sails

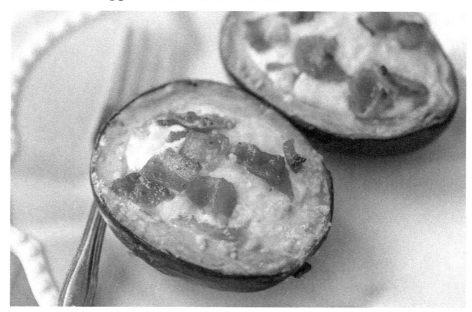

Cook time: 20 mins, Servings 4, Difficulty: easy

Ingredients

- Bacon2½ oz.
- Eggs of large size 2
- Avocado½ (3½ oz.)
- olive oil1 tsp
- Pepper and salt

Instructions

2. Preheat oven to 180°C (350°F). With the help of parchment paper/ foil, line a rimmed baking sheet. Lay the strips of bacon over baking sheet and set them aside.

3. In a saucepan, place the eggs at least 1 inch more than the eggs with cold water. Cover & bring to a slight boil over a high flame. Once the eggs are boiled, take off the pan from the burner and let remaining of the eggs for 15 minutes afterward, covered in the pan. Put eggs to an ice-cold water bowl, using a slotted spoon for about 5-10 minutes, or put them inside colander. Place them under chilled water until they are fully cooled. Peel them, and then set them aside.

4. Inside the middle oven rack, arrange the baking sheet and cook bacon for a duration of 10-20 minutes (time varies with thickness), or till it appears crispy. Dry out bacon over paper towels. When it gets cold, shape the sails.

5. Lengthwise, slice the eggs and scoop the yolks out. In a small bowl, put olive oil, yolks and avocado. The fork is used to mash them until combined. It is then seasoned with salt and pepper to taste.

6. To assemble, spoon out mixture of avocado yolk generously to the egg whites, and arrange bacon sails in the middle of the mixed blend. Cherish and enjoy the unbeatable taste.

Nutrition

Kcal 152, fat 14 g, Protein 6 g, net carbs 1 g

5. Chocolate Keto Protein Shake

Cook time: 5 mins, Servings: 1, Difficulty: easy.

Ingredients

- Almond milk 3/4 c
- Ice1/2 c
- Butter with almonds2 tbsps.
- Cocoa powder (unsweetened) 2 tbsps.
- A sugar substitute for taste such as Swerve 2 - 3 tbsps.
- Seeds of chia can use more for serving1 tbsps.
- Seeds of hemp could use more for serving2 tbsp.
- Vanilla extract (pure form) 1/2 tbsp.
- Pinch kosher salt

Instructions

1. Combine all the blender ingredients and blend until fluffy. Pour chia and hemp seeds for garnishing.

Nutrition

Kcal 440, fat 31.2g g, protein 15.6 g, net carbs 8.2 g

6. Bunless Bacon, Egg & Cheese

Cook time: 10 mins, Servings: 1, Difficulty: easy

Ingredients

- Big eggs2
- Water2 tbsp.
- Avocado, finely mashed1/2
- Cooked slice of bacon, halved 1
- Shredded cheddar1/4 c

Instructions

2. Take two Mason jar lids with centers removed in a medium non-stick pan. The entire pan is to be sprayed with cooking spray and then placed over medium heat. Try to crack the eggs into the centers of the lids and whisk gently to crack the yolk with a fork.

3. Cover the pan by pouring water around the lids. Steam the eggs until the whites are cooked, like for about 3 minutes. Remove the lid. Spread the cheddar on one egg and allow it to cook for about 1 minute so that cheese melts.

4. Turn the side of egg bun onto a tray while not having cheese. Place the avocado and bacon on top. Place the egg bun topped with cheese on top, cheese side down.

Nutrition

Kcal 460, fat 13 g, Protein 27 g, net carbs 8.4 g

7. Avocado Egg Boats

Cook time: 10 mins, Servings: 4, Difficulty: easy

Ingredients

- Avocados (ripe), pitted, and halved2.
- Big eggs4
- Kosher salt
- Ground black pepper (fresh)
- Sliced bacon3
- Fresh chopped chives(garnishing)

Instructions

1. Preheat the oven to 350 degrees. From each half of the avocado, scoop about one tablespoon of avocado. Reserve remaining for another time or discard.

2. In a baking dish, put the hollowed avocados and then crack one egg at a time into the pan. With the help of a spoon, pass yolk to avocado half, using a spoon, and spoon in egg white as you can manage and try not to spill over.

23

3. Bake for about 20 to 25 minutes while seasoning it with salt and pepper until the whites of egg settle down and the yolks are no runnier. (If avocados start to get brown, cover with the foil.)

4. In a bowl over medium flame, cook the bacon for about 8 minutes until it becomes crispy, and then shift it to a plate lined with paper towel. Chop it.

5. When serving, avocados are to be topped with bacon and chives.

Nutrition

Kcal 220, fat 4 g, Protein 6 g, net carbs 7.3 g

8. Loaded Cauliflower Breakfast Bake

Cook time: 15 mins, Servings: 6, Difficulty: easy

Ingredients

- Big cauliflower head1
- Slices of bacon, chopped 8
- Eggs 10
- Whole milk 1 c
- Minced cloves of garlic 2
- Paprika2 tsp
- Kosher salt
- Black pepper
- Crushed cheddar2 c
- Thin sliced green onions, plus more for garnish 2
- Hot sauce to serve

Instructions

1. An oven is preheated to 350 centigrade. On a box grater, grate the head of cauliflower and shift it to a large baking dish.

2. Smoke bacon for about 8 minutes. Inside large skillet medium heat until it becomes crispy. To drain the fat, pass it to a paper towel-lined tray.

3. Whisk the milk, eggs, garlic, and paprika together into a large bowl. Season it with salt and pepper and salt.

4. The cauliflower is topped with cooked bacon, green onions, and cheddar cheese and poured over the egg mixture.

5. This should be baked for 35 to 40 minutes until the eggs are firm and the top gets golden brown in color.

6. It is then garnished with hot sauce and some more green onions.

7. Ready to be served.

Nutrition

Kcal 390, fat 27 g, Protein 28 g, net carbs 6.2 g

9. Spinach Tomato Frittata - Keto

Cook time: 10 mins, Servings: 8, Difficulty: easy

Ingredients

- Big eggs 8
- A cup of spinach 3
- A cup of cherry tomatoes 2
- Bacon chopped slices 8
- Garlic powder 1 tsp
- A cup of cheese (shredded) 1
- Salt
- Black pepper

Instructions

1. First, the oven is preheated to 350 °. A 9-10' deep pie dish is buttered, which is then set aside.

2. Put the bacon on a 12-inch non-stick skillet and cook it on medium-high heat for about 6 to 10 minutes by tossing it frequently until it gets crispy and brown in color.

3. To dry out the bacon, shift it to a plate lined with multiple layers of paper towels. Leave about one tablespoon of bacon fat into the drain of the skillet and reserve or discard excess.

4. Again, put the skillet on a medium-high flame; add on the spinach and tomatoes. Sauté this for about 15 seconds. Move the spinach along with bacon to a plate.

5. Mix well the eggs and garlic powder in a bowl, whisk them until well blended. Now season it with salt and pepper according to taste.

6. Toss the mixture so that ingredients distribute well by adding cooked bacon, spinach, and mozzarella cheese together. Pour this on a dish of the prepared pie.

7. For about 30 – 35 mins, bake it till it settles. It is almost done when a knife inserted in the middle comes out clean. Split into wedges and serve it warm to eat.

Nutrition

Kcal 134, fat 26 g, protein 10 g, net carbs 6 g

Chapter: 3 Bread Recipes

1. The keto bread

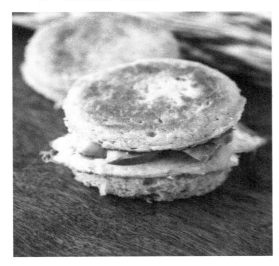

Cook time: 1 hr. +10 mins, Servings: 6, Difficulty: medium

Ingredients

- A cup of ground psyllium husk powder 1/3
- Cups of almond flour 1¼
- Baking powder 2 tsp
- Sea salt 1 tsp
- A cup of water 1
- Cider vinegar 2 tsp
- Egg whites 3
- Sesame seeds 2 tbsp.

Instructions

1. The oven is preheated to 175°C (350°F).

2. In a large mixing bowl, the dry ingredients are mixed. Boil the water.

3. To the dry ingredients, add on vinegar and egg whites, and mix them well. Boiling water is added while beating for approximately 30 seconds with a hand mixer. Don't mix the dough too much; the consistency should be similar to Play-Doh.

4. By applying a little olive oil, moisten the hands. Make six separate rolls from the dough. Place it on a baking sheet that is greased. Top it with sesame seeds (optional).

5. Bake in the oven for 50-60 minutes on the lower rack, based on the bread rolls' size. For confirming, tap the bottom of the bun. A hollow sound could be sensed while tapping the bread, which is an indication that bread is done and is ready to be served.

6. Serve it with butter and toppings depending upon choice.

Nutrition

Kcal 165, fat 12g, Protein 6 g, net carbs 2 g

2. Cheesy Garlic Bread

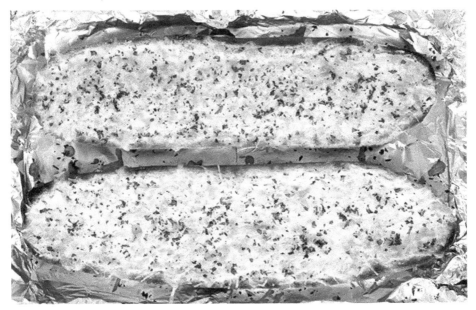

Cook time: 25 mins, Servings: 10, Difficulty: medium

Ingredients

- Bread Base
- Almond flour (Well bee's)1 1/4 C
- Coconut flour 1 T
- Beaten egg whites 3
- Olive oil /avocado oil 2 T
- Lukewarm water 1/4 C
- Yeast (granular form) 1 tsp.
- Coconut sugar (honey)1 tsp
- Mozzarella cheese (shredded) 1/2 C
- Salt 1/4 tsp
- Baking powder 2 tsp.

- Garlic powder 1/4 tsp.
- Xanthan gum (optional) 1/2 tsp.

Topping

- A cup of mozzarella cheese(shredded) 1
- Melted butter 2 T
- Garlic powder 1/4 tsp.
- Salt 1/4 tsp.
- Italian seasoning 1/2 tsp.

Instructions

1. Preheat the oven to 400°C.
2. Mix coconut flour, almond, salt, baking powder, garlic powder, and xanthan gum together in a large cup. Stir them all well.
3. Add warm water and sugar to a shallow bowl. Stir them to dissolve, and then add yeast. Leave it aside for a few mins.
4. With the help of a rubber spatula, apply olive oil and yeast-water mixture to the flour mixture, and then stir it with the help of a rubber spatula. Add on beaten eggs while mixing.
5. Mozzarella shreds 1/2 Care added to the mixture with gentle mixing using a spatula until the cheese is well combined and pleasant dough is formed.
6. Grease a 9-9 square cake pan or large sheet of cookies. Pour the batter onto a cookie sheet or cake pan. On the cookie sheet, loosely shape the dough into a rectangle or square.
7. Bake at about 400 degrees, approximately for 15-17 mins or until the crust sides turn golden brown. Now remove it and top.
8. Just mix the butter, garlic powder, and salt in a tiny bowl and brush over the base of the garlic bread. Make sure the butter gets over every inch.
9. Place the shredded mozzarella cheese on top of the bread, and then sprinkle it with Italian seasoning.

10. Bake it for 10 minutes at 400 degrees, or till the cheese melts. Turn on the broiler for the final 3 minutes to brown the cheese.

11. Take away the bread from the oven and allow it to stand before serving for 5-10 minutes.

Nutrition

Kcal 175, fat 16g, Protein 8 g, net carbs 4 g

3. Almond Buns

Cook time: 15 mins, Servings: 3, Difficulty: easy

Ingredients

- Cups of Bob's Red Mill Almond Flour ¾ cup
- Big Eggs 2
- Unsalted Butter5 Tbsp.
- Splenda (optional)1.5 tsp
- Baking Powder1.5 tsp

Instructions

1. Put the dry ingredients in a bowl and blend.
2. Whisk the eggs together.
3. Melt the butter, blend and whisk in the mixture.
4. Divide the mixture into six sections equally in a Muffin Top tray.
5. Bake it in an oven at 350 degrees for 12–17 minutes.
6. Just allow it cool on a wire rack.

Nutrition

Kcal 373, fat 35g, protein 12 g, net carbs 7.2 g

4. Keto fathead pizza

Cook time: 20 mins, Servings: 8 slices, Difficulty: easy

Ingredients

- A cup of shredded Mozzarella cheese 2 cups

- Cream cheese 2 tbsp.

- Almond Flour 1 cup

- Large egg 1

- Baking powder 1 tsp

- Italian seasoning(optional) 1 tsp

- Garlic powder (optional) 1 tsp

- Toppings

- Fresh mozzarella/ parmesan.

- Pepperoni, turkey.

- Jalapeno/pepper/olives/ spinach.

- Sugar-free tomato sauce/ blue cheese, and buffalo.

- Crushed Red Peppers

Instructions

1. An oven is preheated to 450F.

2. Add cream cheese and mozzarella to a sizeable bowl and microwave them for 45 seconds.

3. After removing from the microwave, add in the egg, garlic, almond flour, baking powder, and Italian seasoning. Mix until well blended, with a spoon.

4. The dough is shifted onto a large piece of parchment paper while covering it with another piece of paper. Flatten the dough to around 1/4 "thick using a rolling pin. Remove the parchment paper and shape it with your hands if necessary.

5. Shift the pizza on a baking sheet or pizza stone over the parchment paper and bake it for 10 minutes.

6. While keeping the oven on, remove the pizza. Serve with all of your favorite sauces and toppings.

7. Bake pizza for another 5-8 minutes or until the cheese is bubbly.

Nutrition

Kcal 249, fat 19g, Protein 14g, net carbs 6.8 g

5. Keto pizza

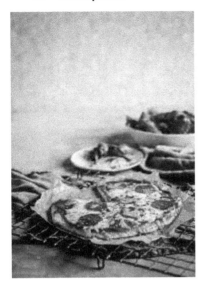

Cook time: 25 mins, Servings: 2 slices, Difficulty: medium

Ingredients

- Crust
- Eggs 4
- Mozzarella cheese (shredded) 1½ cups
- Topping
- Tomato sauce (unsweetened) 3 tbsp.
- Oregano(dried) 1 tsp
- Provolone shredded cheese1¼ cups
- Pepperoni 1½ oz.
- Olives (optional)

For serving

- Leafy greens 1 cup
- A cup of olive oil¼

- Salt
- Black pepper (grounded)

Instructions

1. Preheat the oven to 200 centigrade.

2. Begin by forming the crust. Crack the eggs and add the shredded cheese to a medium-sized dish. Stir it well so that it mixes properly.

3. The baking sheet is lined with parchment paper for spreading the cheese and egg batter. It can be formed in any shape, either form two round circles or just make one big rectangular pizza. Bake for 15 minutes in the oven until the crust of the pizza turns golden. Remove and leave for a minute or two to cool.

4. Raise the temperature of the oven is to 225°C (450°F).

5. Spread the tomato sauce on the crust and top it with sprinkled oregano, some more cheese, pepperoni, and olives on top.

6. Bake it for a time of about 5-10 minutes or until the brown color of the pizza has turned golden.

7. Balance and serve it with a fresh salad.

Nutrition

Kcal 1024, fat 86g, Protein 56g, net carbs 6 g

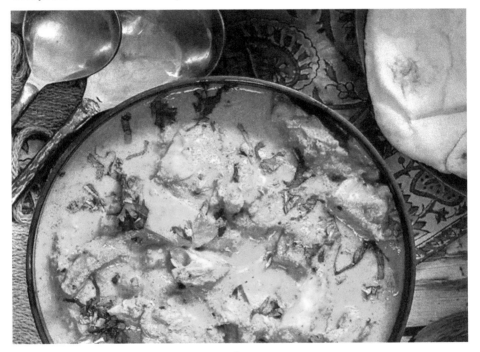

1. **Low-carb butter chicken salad**

Cook time: 20-25 mins, Servings: 4, Difficulty: easy.

Ingredients

- A cup of Greek yogurt ¾
- Tandoori paste 2½ tbsp.
- Vegetable oil 1 tbsp.

- Garam masala 2½tsp.
- Lily dale Free Range Thigh of Chicken 8
- Red onion, thin slices 1
- Juice of lemon 1
- Caster sugar ¼ tsp.
- Lebanese cucumber, sliced in round shape 1
- Tomatoes small truss halved 250g
- Green chilies (sliced) 2
- Curry leaves chopped 2 tbsp. (optional)
- A big bunch of coriander leaves 1
- A cup of chopped roasted cashews⅓ cup

Instructions

1. In a baking dish, mix 1/4 cup (70g) yogurt, 1 1/2 tbsp. tandoori paste, 1 tbsp. Olive oil and 2 tsp. garam masala, and set it aside.

2. Place two thighs of chicken on a cutting board. To make three separate skewers, pass three skewers through the thighs, and then cut them parallel to the middle skewer. To make 12 skewers, repeat the step. Marinade the skewers to toss until fully covered, using your fingertips. Take at least 30 minutes.

3. Preheat the oven grill and set a shelf in the oven in a lower position. Cover a second baking dish with foil, narrower than the length of the skewers. Place skewers over the prepared dish so that the chicken settles above the dish's surface. Grill it for 10 minutes till slightly charred. Turn the side and grill for an additional 5-10 minutes.

4. In the meantime, in a cup, combine the onion, lemon juice, 1 tsp. Salt, sugar, and the rest of 1/2 tsp. garam masala and shake to blend. Set aside until necessary. Place the cucumber, chili, curry leaves and cilantro in a bowl and set aside until appropriate.

36

5. Combine in a bowl the remaining 1/2 cup of yogurt and 1 tbsp. All of them are combined to create a swirl effect with a spoon. For cucumber salad, drained pickled onion is added and tossed until well blended. Assemble it on serving plates. Sprinkle over some of the cooking juices. Then add skewers to the dishes. Scatter with cashews and chili leftovers to serve.

Nutrition

Kcal 122, fat 8.7g, protein 10.2g, net carbs 2.6 g

2. Yogurt and lime grilled chicken

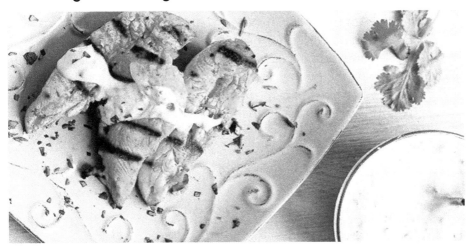

Cook time: 40 mins, Servings: 4, Difficulty: capable.

Ingredient

- Lily dale Free Range Whole Chicken 1.6kg

- A cup of ras el hanout (Moroccan spice) quarter of cup

- Greek-style yoghurt(thick) 1 cup

- Juice of lemon 1

- Virgin olive oil 2 tbsp.

- Lime wedges

Instructions

1. Take breast and leg, slice two shallow slits, and then sprinkle salt flakes all over the chicken.

2. In a big bowl, mix yogurt, ras el hanout, lemon juice, and 1 tsp of salt. Put the chicken and then turn it well to coat. To marinate, chill for a minimum of 2 hours or let it stay overnight.

3. Preheat on a medium-high pan with chargrill and oven it to 180 degrees Celsius. Now pick out the chicken from the fridge 30 minutes before cooking. Take out the chicken from the marinade, allowing the excess to slip away. Glaze with oil and cook for 5 minutes until it turns golden. Turn and cook, or until golden, for another 5 minutes. Shift it to a baking tray by doing the breast side up and then roast in the oven for 30-40 minutes till the juices start appearing clear when the thigh is pierced with a skewer. In the meantime, close the barbecue hood and reduce the heat to a medium amount. Cook it for about 30-40 minutes. Let it rest for 10 minutes while loosely covered with foil

4. The grilled chicken is then seasoned with salt and served with lime.

Nutrition

Kcal 134, fat 9.4g, protein 10g, net carbs 0.8 g

3. Simple keto meatballs

Cook time: 20 mins, Servings: 1, Difficulty: easy

Ingredients

- Beef (grounded) 1 lb.
- Eggs 1
- A cup of grated parmesan half cup
- A cup of shredded mozzarella half cup
- Garlic (minced) 1 tbsp.
- Blackpepper1 tsp.
- Salt1/2 tsp.
- Perfect keto unflavored whey protein (optional)1 scoop

Instructions

1. Firstly, line the baking sheet with parchment paper by preheating the oven to 400 degrees.

2. Add all the ingredients to a bowl and mix them with the help of your hands and knead until everything is nicely incorporated.

3. Take the mixture and make meatballs of the same size and position them on the prepared baking sheet.

4. Bake it for 18-20 minutes, then.

5. Allow it to cool

6. Serve warm.

Nutrition

Kcal 153, fat 10.9g, protein 12.2g,net carbs 0.7 g

4. Creamy Tuscan garlic butter shrimp

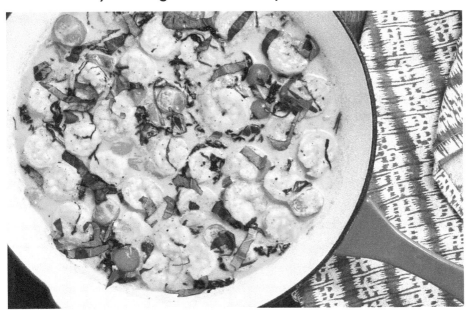

Cook time: 15 mins, Servings: 6, Difficulty: easy

Ingredients

- Butter 2 tbsp.

- Tail-off white medium-sized shrimp (cooked) 2 pounds
- Onion, (small and diced)¼
- Red bell pepper(diced/ chopped) 1
- Cloves garlic(minced) 4-6
- Canned full-fat coconut milk (one/ 13.5 ounce)
- Spinach /kale 2 cups
- Grated parmesan cheese(one/ 5-ounce container)
- Perfect keto unflavouredcollagen3 scoops
- Sea salt 1tsp
- Black pepper 1tsp
- Italian seasoning 1tbsp

Instructions

1. Add on the red bell pepper, shrimp, butter, onion, and minced garlic to large stainless steel over medium-high heat, stir it to combine, and cook until the onions appear translucent in color for around 6-8 minutes.

2. Add coconut milk / heavy cream, sea salt, spinach, pepper, parmesan cheese, and seasoning. Stir them all to mix and bring to a boil.

3. Turn down the heat to medium-low and leave for 15 minutes to simmer.

4. Top it with finely chopped parsley over cauliflower rice or steamed broccoli.

Nutrition

Kcal 334, fat 15.8g, Protein 27.25g, net carbs4 g

5. Keto creamy garlic lemon zucchini pasta

Cook time: 10 mins, Servings: 2, Difficulty: easy

Ingredients

- Zucchini noodles two large

- Olive oil 2tbsp
- Lemon 1 (zest reserved + 1/3 cup of fresh lemon juice)
- Clove of garlic finely minced four cloves.
- Salt½tsp
- Black pepper¼tp
- Cream cup ¼
- Fresh basil/ parsley (a handful of roughly chopped)

Instructions

1. In a large saucepan set over medium heat, add olive oil.
2. Continue cooking by adding garlic for 30 seconds until you could smell the aroma.
3. In the pan, add on with the lemon juice and zest along with salt, pepper, and heavy cream. Cook for 8-10 minutes to minimize the sauce. Adjust the seasoning according to taste. Turn the heat off.
4. Now add on zucchini noodles in it, and then toss in the sauce.
5. Serve it with parmesan chicken or mini meatloaves as an aside. Use herbs for garnishing. Enjoy the meal.

Nutrition

Kcal 283, fat 25g, Protein 4g, net carbs 12 g

6. Keto crescent rolls

Cook time: 30 mins, Servings: 8, Difficulty: medium

Ingredients

Mozzarella cheese4 oz

- Cream cheese(shredded) 2 oz
- Egg 1
- Almond flour cup 1 cup
- Coconut flour cup ¼ cup

- Monk fruit 1tbsp

- Baking powder 1 tsp

- Salt¼ tsp

Instructions

1. In a heat-proof container, add mozzarella and cream cheese. Microwave at intervals of 30 seconds until completely melted.

2. Now whisk the egg and pour into the mixture of cheese.

3. Then add the monk fruit, almond flour, coconut flour, baking powder, and salt to a separate bowl. Whisk in order to combine.

4. Blend wet and dry ingredients together with the spoon.

5. Knead and shape the dough into a small ball. Enroll in a wrap of plastic and cool for 20-30 minutes.

6. An oven is now preheated to 350 °F. Parchment paper is used to line a baking pan.

7. The dough is now taken out of the refrigerator, and the plastic is removed. Press the dough into a rectangular shape using a rolling pin.

8. Shape into a triangle (large end to small end). Roll them to create the classic "crescent roll."

9. Bake them for 20- 25 minutes until they get the golden brown.

Nutrition

Kcal 147, fat 11g, Protein 8g, net carbs 12 g

7. Keto parmesan chicken

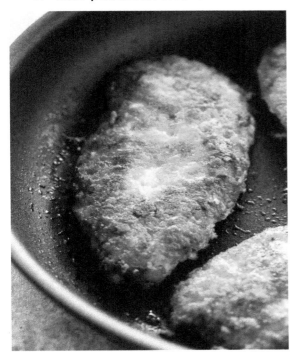

Cook time: 30 mins, Servings: 4, Difficulty: medium.

Ingredients

- Chicken breasts4–6
- Egg 1
- A cup of almond flour¾ cup
- A grated cup of parmesan cheese¼ cup
- Salt1 ½ tsp
- Black pepper ¼ tsp
- Garlic powder1 tbsp.
- Italian seasoning 2 tsp
- Olive oil 1 tbsp.
- A cup of broccoli florets2 cups

43

- Salt ½ tsp
- Marinara sauce cup ¼ cup
- Extra parmesan cheese

Instructions

1. The first oven is preheated to 400°. The oven is lined with a baking sheet along with parchment paper. It is then set aside.

2. To a clean shallow bowl, add almond flour, pepper, and parmesan cheese, 1 tsp of salt, garlic powder, and Italian seasoning. Mix all the ingredients well. In a separate dish, add an egg and whisk well.

3. Coat the egg mixture on chicken breasts and then with the almond flour mixture. Set it up in the baking pan.

4. Bake it in the oven for almost 10 minutes. Now remove it from the oven. Just add broccoli. Drizzle some olive oil and the remaining 1/2 tsp of salt over broccoli. Toss it well to coat it. Add on extra parmesan cheese and marinara sauce on top of chicken breast.

5. Again place the pan into the oven for an added 10 minutes until the chicken gets cooked. Cooking time can differ depending on chicken thickness.

Nutrition

Kcal 273, fat 14g, protein 33g,net carbs 14 g

Chapter 5: Drink recipes

1. Green turmeric tea

Cook time: 5 mins, Servings: 1 cup, Difficulty: easy

Ingredients

- Almond milk(warmed)1¼ cup
- Perfect keto matcha(MCT oil powder)1 scoop
- Cinnamon½ tsp.
- Ground turmeric½–¼ tsp.
- Black pepper (grounded) ¼ tsp.
- Ginger ¼ tsp.
- vanilla flavoring(non-alcoholic) 1 teaspoon
- Stevia/ monk fruit sweetener to taste (optional)

Instructions

1. To a high-speed blender, combine all the ingredients and blend till all the ingredients just mix well.

Nutrition

Kcal 107.5, fat 10.1g, Protein 1g, net carbs 1.5 g

2. Keto protein shake

Cook time: 5 mins, Servings: 1 cup, Difficulty: easy

Ingredients

- Almond milk(unsweetened) 1 cup
- A cup of full-fat coconut milk/ heavy cream 1/4 cup
- Perfect keto chocolate whey protein powder one scoop
- Cacao powder 2 tsp
- Liquid stevia 8–10 drops
- Perfect keto nut butter/ almond butter one teaspoon
- Ice cubes 3–4

- Cacao nibs (optional) 1 tablespoon
- Whipped cream (optional) 2 tablespoons

Instructions

1. Place all the ingredients together and blend until they appear smooth.
2. If preferred, top with Perfect Keto Nut Butter or almond butter, cacao nibs, flakes of coconut, or nuts.

Nutrition

Kcal 273, fat 20g, Protein 17g, net carbs 1.7 g

3. Keto Birthday Cake Shake

Cook time: 5 mins, Servings: 2 cups, Difficulty: easy

Ingredients

- A cup of heavy cream ¼ cup
- A cup of nut milk 1½ cup
- Butter 1tbsp
- Vanilla extract 2 tsp
- Perfect Keto Birthday Cake bar 1
- Swerve/ Lakanto/ keto-friendly sweetener of choice to taste
- Ice (handful)
- Topping(sugar-free sprinkles)

Instructions

1. Add all the required ingredients to a high-speed blender and blend it at high speed until all the ingredients are mixed well.

Nutrition

Kcal 291.3, fat 26.8g, Protein 7.25g, net carbs 3.5 g

4. Chocolate peanut butter smoothie

Cook time: 5 mins, Servings: 2 cups, Difficulty: easy

Ingredients

- almond milk(unsweetened) / low-carb, plant-based milk 1 cup (240 ml)
- creamy peanut butter 2tbsp (32g)
- cocoa powder(unsweetened) 1tbsp(4g)
- heavy cream cup 1/4 cup (60 ml)
- a cup of ice 1

Instructions

1. Blend to combine and mix the ingredients in a blender until smooth.

Nutrition

Kcal 345, fat 31g, Protein 11g, net carbs 13 g

5. Coconut blackberry mint smoothie

Cook time: 5 mins, Servings: 1 cup, Difficulty: easy

Ingredients

- Full-fat coconut milk(unsweetened) 1/2 cup
- A cup of frozen blackberries 1/2 cup
- Shredded coconut 2tbsp
- Mint leaves 5-10 leaves

Instructions

1. In a blender, combine and blend until smooth and fluffy.

Nutrition

Kcal 321, fat 29g, Protein 4g, net carbs 17 g

6. Strawberries and cream smoothie

Cook time: 5 mins, Servings: 1 cup, Difficulty: easy

Ingredients

- Water 1/2 cup

- Strawberries froze 1/2 cup
- Heavy cream 1/2 cup

Instructions

1. Take all the ingredients; combine them in a blender until smooth.

Nutrition

Kcal 431, fat 43g, Protein 4g, net carbs 10 g

7. Pumpkin spice smoothie

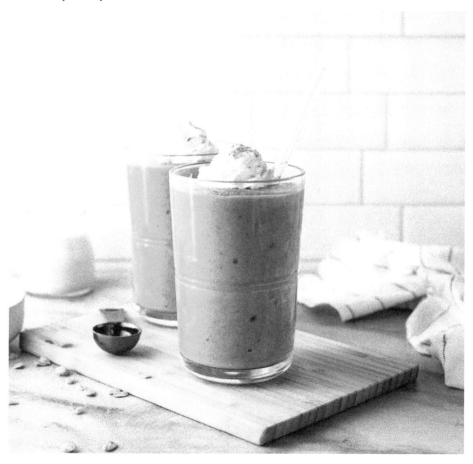

Cook time: 5 mins, Servings: 1 cup, Difficulty: easy

Ingredients

- Unsweetened coconut(unsweetened) / almond milk 1/2 cup
- Pumpkin purée 1/2 cup
- Almond butter 2tbsp
- Pumpkin pie spice ¼ tsp
- A cup of ice 1/2
- Pinch of sea salt

Instructions

1. Take all the ingredients; combine them in a blender until smooth and fluffy.

Nutrition

Kcal 462, fat 42g, Protein 10g, net carbs 19 g

Chapter 6: Vegetable Recipes

1. Mashed Cauliflower with Parmesan and Chives

Cook time: 20 mins, Servings: 4-6 cups, Difficulty: easy

Ingredients

- Small heads cauliflower (cored and leaves removed)2 heads
- Chicken broth 2 cups
- Parmesan cheese(grated) 1/4 cup
- Chopped chives (fresh) 1/4 cup
- Kosher salt
- Fresh ground black pepper

Instructions

1. Add the cauliflower and chicken broth to a medium-sized saucepan, give it a boil. Reduce heat to low. Cover the saucepan and cook for 15 - 20 minutes until the cauliflower becomes tender.

2. Afterward, with the help of a slotted spoon, shift the cauliflower to a food processor and purée until smooth.

3. This mixture is then shifted to a bowl and stirred in parmesan and chopped chives. Season it with kosher salt and fresh ground black pepper. Serve it sweet.

Nutrition

Kcal 33, fat 2g, Protein 3g, net carbs 1 g

2. Curry roasted cauliflower

Cook time: 15 mins, Servings: 4, Difficulty: easy

Ingredients

- Cauliflower(about 2 pounds) 1 head
- Virgin olive oil 1 tbsp. + 1 tsp extra
- Curry powder one ½tsp

- Kosher salt 1tsp
- Lemon juice 2tsp
- Chopped cilantro 1tbsp (to taste)

Instructions

1. First, the oven is preheated to 425° F.

2. Cutaway the outer cauliflower leaves. Split it in half and then cut out and discard the core, which is left out. Slice the cauliflower into parts that are bite-sized. In a deep bowl, cauliflower is tossed with olive oil to coat. Sprinkle with curry powder and salt and cover with a toss. It is then spread out as evenly layered on a large lined and moved into the oven.

3. Roast the cauliflower for about 10 minutes before the bottom starts to tan. Flip it over and continue roasting for more than 5 to 7 minutes till tender. Squeeze the lemon juice and cilantro and toss it all.

Nutrition

Kcal 110, fat 8g, Protein 3g, net carbs 8 g

3. Cauliflower Steaks (roasted) served with Caper M Butter

Cook time: 25 mins, Servings: 4, Difficulty: easy

Ingredients

- Cauliflower (cut into steaks) 1 large head
- Olive oil (as needed) 3-4 tbsp
- Freshly ground black pepper.
- Salt
- Mustard caper browned butter.
- Unsalted butter one stick
- Cloves of garlic(minced) 2
- Coarse-grain mustard 2tbsp
- Drained capers 2tbsp

- Chopped parsley 2tbsp
- Salt
- Ground black pepper(to taste)

Instructions

Cauliflower:

1. To 400 °, the oven is preheated.
2. Over a non-stick baking sheet or aluminum foil, place cauliflower florets or steaks.
3. Brush the cauliflower with olive oil and season properly with salt and black pepper. Let it roast for about 20-25 minutes, turning once.

Brown butter:

1. Butter is placed and melted over medium flame in a saucepan.
2. Reduce the flame and cook for about 5 minutes until caramel color starts appearing, taking care not to burn it.
3. Place it aside now so that the browned bits (milk solids) fall at the end of the pan.
4. Stir in capers, garlic, chopped parsley, mustard. Add to taste, salt, and pepper. Sprinkle over roasted cauliflower and serve warm.
5. It is possible to make butter up to 24 hours in advance. Refrigerate and cool. Reheat gently over low heat in a saucepan.

Nutrition

Kcal 592, fat 8g, Protein 22 g, net carbs 16 g

4. **Roasted Vegetables with combination of Moroccan Cauliflower Rice**

Cook Time: 50 mins, Servings: 4, Difficulty: capable

Ingredients

- Cauliflower 1

- Mixed peppers(green, yellow, red, and sliced) 3
- Sliced courgettes zucchini 2
- Sliced aubergine 1
- Chopped spring onions 2
- A crushed clove of garlic 1
- Red chili (chopped) 1
- Cumin(grounded) 1 tsp
- Pistachios (roasted) handful
- Parsley(chopped) 50g
- Chopped mint 50g
- A cup of full fat natural yoghurt1/2 cup
- Tahini 2 tbsp.
- Lemon (unwaxed) 1

Instructions

1. First, simply oven is heated to 200 Celsius in advance.
2. Now we slice the peppers, aubergine, and courgettes, leaving back 1/2 red pepper that is thinly sliced and will go into the cauliflower rice.
3. Put in olive oil, toss it, and then add salt and roast for 45-50 minutes. Turn around halfway through.
4. Dry-roast the pistachios now. Simply place them over medium heat in a pan and roast until they are browned. This may take 2 minutes or so. Be careful they aren't burning.
5. Simply blend 150g / 1/2 cup yogurt with two tablespoons of tahini and 1/2 lemon juice in order to make the yogurt tahini sauce. Add a bit of garlic, too, if you like.
6. To make rice for cauliflower, cut off all the outer leaves and the cauliflower into pieces. Cut the rough center out. Next, in the food processor, grate or blitz large chunks until you get rice-sized bits.

7. In a saucepan, just heat one tablespoon of olive oil and add garlic which has been crushed, spring onions nicely chopped, the finely chopped half pepper, and the chopped chili. For 2 minutes, cook it gently.

8. Now add the cauliflower and cook for an additional 5 minutes.

9. Stir in 1 tablespoon of cumin, 1/2 lemon juice, and lemon zest, and also the dry-roasted pistachios.

10. Remove the cauliflower rice from the flame. Now add on the parsley and mint before serving, and combine thoroughly. Add few scattered pomegranate seeds if desired.

11. Organize on one large platter or serve the veggies and rice separately on two plates.

12. The dish tastes pretty good, hot or cold.

Nutrition

Kcal 147, fat 7.4g, Protein 6.8g, net carbs 17.8 g

5. Cauliflower rice with garlic and green onion

Cook time: 30 mins, Servings: 4, Difficulty: easy

Ingredients

- Cauliflower pieces(stems included) 4 heaping cups
- Olive oil2 t
- Cloves of garlic(cut in half) big eight cloves
- Sliced green onion 1 cup
- Salt(to taste)
- Black pepper (fresh and grounded to taste)
- For using a 12 oz. Bag of riced cauliflower
- Riced cauliflower 12 oz.
- Olive oil 1 1/2 t
- Cloves of garlic 5-6
- Green onion(sliced) 3/4 cup

- Salt (to taste)
- Fresh black pepper (to taste)

Instructions

1. Slice the cauliflower into smaller pieces of the same size until four generous cups of pieces of cauliflower, including the stems, are ready.

2. Process 2 cups of cauliflower pieces at the moment in the food processor using the steel blade, buzzing it in short bursts until it is finely chopped enough, but slightly larger, to resemble rice.

3. Open the bag of cauliflower if available.

4. The garlic cloves are peeled and then slice them lengthwise in half.

5. Chop sufficient green onions for the amount of cauliflower we have.

6. Oil is heated over a low flame in a non-stick frying pan until it feels hot, then put the garlic cloves and stir-fry until garlic smell could be sensed.

7. The moment there is the slightest color change in the garlic, remove the garlic and discard.

8. Now put the cauliflower in the hot pan while season it with salt and freshly ground black pepper.

9. Fry the cauliflower and turn it over regularly until it starts to soften and lose the raw flavor, around 3-4 minutes.

10. Turn off the flame, add the green onions, and serve right away.

Nutrition

Kcal 181, fat 13g, Protein 5g, net carbs 7.6 g

6. Cauliflower Cheese & Onion Croquette

Cook time: 15 mins, servings: 12 croquettes, Difficulty: medium

Ingredients

- Cauliflower 1

- parmesan cheese (grated) 1 cup
- Garlic powder 2tsp
- Spring onions(chopped) 4
- Cheddar cheese grated 1/2 cup
- Dijon mustard1/2 tsp
- Salt ½ tsp
- Pepper ½ tsp
- Olive oil 2tbsp

Instructions

1. First, the cauliflower is chopped into florets, put in a water pan, bring it to a boil, cover, and simmer until soft for 10-15 minutes.
2. Now drain the water and let it cool.
3. Draw out the excess water from the florets by squeezing.
4. Mash the cauliflower by using a hand or with a blender.
5. Add the remaining spring onions, 1 cup of Parmesan cheese, Cheddar cheese, mustard, and seasoning. Thoroughly blend.
6. Make croquettes shapes by using your hand.
7. Layer the croquettes on parchment/greaseproof paper and place them in the refrigerator for about 30 minutes.
8. Now on a frying pan, heat the olive oil over a medium flame.
9. Fry the croquettes softly, turning over until the color is golden.
10. Ready to eat and enjoy.

Nutrition

Kcal 86, fat 6g, Protein 5g, net carbs 2.6 g

7. Roasted Garlic-Parmesan Zucchini, Squash, and Tomatoes

Cook time: 30 mins, Servings: 6 servings, Difficulty: medium

Ingredients

- Small zucchini (half an inch thick slices) 2

- Yellow squash (small sized) (half an inch slice) 2

- Flavoring /small tomatoes (Campari) 14 oz

- Olive oil 3tbp

- Minced cloves of garlic 4

- Italian seasoning one and a half tsp

- Salt and black pepper(grounded)

- Shredded parmesan cheese a full cup(2.4 oz)

- Fresh/ parsley dried (for garnish)

Instructions

1. First, we preheat the oven to a temperature of 400 °. Line the oven with an 18 by 13-inch rimmed baking sheet along with aluminum foil or a sheet of parchment paper. Altogether whisk the garlic, olive oil, and also the remaining Italian seasoning in a bowl (let it rest for a time of 5 - 10 minutes if possible so that flavors absorb into oil). In another bowl, put the zucchini, tomatoes and squash altogether. Pour the mixture of olive oil over the top and toss gently with your hands to blend evenly.

2. Pour onto a fully prepared baking dish and distribute it evenly. With the combination of salt and some amount of pepper, season it. Sprinkle each top with parmesan. Roast 25 - 30 minutes in a preheated oven till the veggies are soft and tender, and the parmesan gets golden brown in color. If desired, garnish it with some parsley and serve hot.

Nutrition

Kcal 168, fat 11g, Protein 5g, net carbs 8 g

8. Bacon & smoked gouda cauliflower mash (low carb and gluten free)

Cook time: 20 mins, Servings: 3 cups, Difficulty: easy

Ingredients

- Cauliflower florets 4 cups
- Heavy cream 3tbsp
- Butter 2tbsp
- Kosher salt 1/2 tsp
- Black pepper 1/4 tsp
- Garlic powder 1/4 tsp
- Cooked bacon four slices
- Smoked gouda cheese(shredded) 1/3 cup
- Salt (to taste)
- Pepper(to taste)

Instructions

1. In the microwave dish, the cauliflower, garlic powder, heavy cream, butter, salt, and pepper are placed. Microwave them all for 18 to 20 minutes until soft. Move the liquid and cauliflower to a food processor. Further, add the bacon and the smoked Gouda in it. Blend until creamy and smooth. As needed, season with additional pinch of salt and some pepper

Nutrition

Kcal 282, fat 22g, Protein 12g, net carbs 6 g

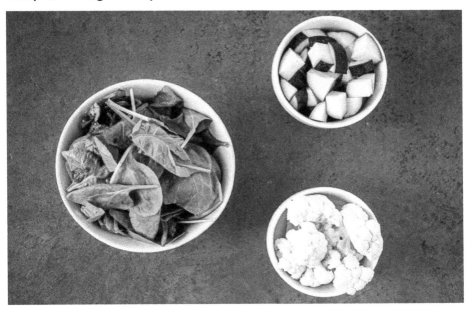

1. **Smoothie Bowl (low carb) with Cauliflower and Greens**

Cook time: 15 mins, Servings: 2, Difficulty: easy

Ingredients

- Frozen cauliflower1/2 cup
- Frozen zucchini1/2 cup
- Frozen spinach 1 cup
- Frozen blueberries 1 cup
- A cup of milk 1 cup
- Almond butter/peanut butter2 tbsp
- Hemp hearts3 tbsp
- Cinnamon (grounded)1 tsp
- Optional toppings
- Berries (fresh /frozen)
- Granola (grain-free)

Instructions

1. This bowl of smoothie fits best with frozen cauliflower and zucchini. The choice of steaming the cauliflower first, but this move is not required when using a high-speed blender such as a Vitamix. It's convenient to have frozen spinach, but fresh works fine as well.

2. We combine all of the ingredients in a blender, beginning with the frozen ingredients close to the blade. Blend till a creamy consistency is obtained and all the ingredients are well integrated.

3. The banana-free smoothie bowl mix should be split into two bowls. Homemade granola, new fruit, and extra hemp hearts are used for topping.

4. Try to steam a big batch of it in the freezer and store it.

Nutrition

Kcal 253, fat 14.8g, Protein 12g, net carbs 18.5 g

2. Best ever guacamole

Cook time: 10 mins, Servings: 4, Difficulty: easy

Ingredients

- Avocados(ripe) 3
- Onion(small and finely diced) 1/2
- Roma tomatoes(nicely diced) 2
- Fresh cilantro(chopped) 3tbsp
- Jalapeno pepper(seeds removed) 1
- Garlic cloves(minced) 2 cloves
- Lime(juiced) 1
- Sea salt ½ tsp

Instructions

1. In a large bowl, chop the avocados in half, remove out the pit and scoop out.

2. Avocado is scooped into a mixing bowl.

3. With the help of a fork, avocado is mashed, and it is made as chunky or smooth as you would like.

4. Mix and stir together the remaining ingredients. Try giving it a taste test and, if necessary, add a little bit more salt or lime juice.

5. Now plate the guacamole with tortilla chips.

6. Guacamole next to tortilla chips is served.

Nutrition

Kcal 184.8, fat 15.8g, Protein 2.5g, net carbs 12.3 g

3. Maple low carb oatmeal

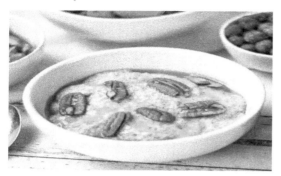

Cook Time: 20 mins, Servings: 4, Difficulty: easy

Ingredients

- Walnuts(1/2 cups)
- Pecans(1/2 cups)
- Sunflower seeds (1/4 cups)
- Coconut flakes (1/4 cups)
- Almond milk(unsweetened) 4 cups
- Chia seeds 4tbsp
- Stevia powder3/8 tsp
- Cinnamon1/2 tsp
- maple flavoring (optional)1 tsp

Instructions

1. In a food processor, add the walnuts, sunflower seeds, and pecans and pulse them a few times to crumble.

2. Add all of the ingredients into a big pot. Stir on low and simmer for a reasonable 20-30 minutes, until most of the liquid has been absorbed by the chia seeds. Don't forget to stir, as the seeds will stick to the bottom of the jar.

3. Turn down the heat when the oatmeal appears thickened and serve warm. It can also be cooled down and stored the next day in the refrigerator for breakfast.

4. End up serving with fresh fruit and any other toppings needed.

Nutrition

Kcal 374, fat 34.59g, Protein 9.25g, net carbs 3.274 g

4. Vegan Arugula Avocado Tomato Salad

Cook time: 20 mins, Servings: 8, Difficulty: easy

Ingredients

- Arugula Salad
- Baby arugula(chopped roughly) 5 oz
- Large basil leaves (sliced) 6 leaves
- Pint yellow grape tomatoes half sliced.
- Pint red grape tomatoes half sliced.
- Large avocados(chunks) 2
- Red onion (minced) 1/2 cup
- Balsamic Vinaigrette
- Balsamic vinegar 2 tbsp
- Olive oil 1tbsp
- Maple syrup 1 tbsp
- Juice of lemon 1 tbsp
- Garlic clove(minced) 1
- Himalayan pink sea salt 1/4 tsp
- Black pepper 1/4 tsp

Instructions

1. Put the roughly chopped arugula and sliced basil leaves into a large mixing bowl. Add the sliced grape tomatoes, avocado chunks, and minced red onion to the bowl. Toss to combine.

2. Put into a large mixing bowl the finely chopped arugula and basil leaves which have been sliced. Add to the bowl the sliced grape tomatoes, chunks of avocado, and minced red onion. Now toss it to combine.

3. Now the balsamic dressing is poured over the salad. Mix the salad carefully until the dressing is uniformly distributed, and then moves the salad to a large bowl.

Note

- Chop the arugula roughly so it is bite-sized.

- Wait until you serve to add the avocado if you are making this vegan arugula salad to bring to a dinner. If the avocado chunks are added too early, they may begin to turn brown. Add few drops of lemon juice over the avocado chunks if you have to add the avocado early to prevent them from turning brown.

- For this salad, use avocados that are firm with only a little bit of giving when pressing them. If the avocado is sufficiently soft for guacamole, then this is too ripe for the dish. Avocado should retain its shape when tossed.

- If the avocados are a little soft, dice them instead of mixing them into the salad and top the salad with them. This way, once you toss it, the avocado will not break down and become too mushy in the salad.

- Store it for 1-2 days in an airtight jar in the fridge if there is some leftover arugula salad. The next day, that salad won't be as fresh, but it would still be edible. When about to eat it, add a little bit of fresh arugula to the leftovers to freshen it up.

Nutrition

Kcal 134, fat 9g, Protein 3g, net carbs 12 g

5. Vegan Sesame Ginger Coleslaw

Cook time: 15 mins, Servings: 12 servings, Difficulty: easy

Ingredients

- Sesame Ginger Dressing -
- Almond butter2 tbsp.
- Tahini 1tbsp.
- Low-sodium tamari2 tbsp.
- Rice vinegar2 tbsp.
- Lime (juice) 3tbsp.
- Hot sauce 1tbsp.
- Maple syrup 1tbsp.
- Medium clove of garlic (peeled) 1
- Fresh ginger (peeled) 2-inch knob

Coleslaw -

- Green cabbage(sliced thinly) 5 cups
- Red cabbage(sliced thinly) 5 cups
- Carrots (sliced thinly) 2 cups
- Cilantro (roughly chopped) 1 cup
- Green onions (sliced) 1 cup

Instructions

1. Put two tablespoons of almond butter, one tablespoon of tahini, two tablespoons of rice vinegar, two tablespoons of tamari, three tablespoons of lime juice, one tablespoon of hot sauce, one tablespoon of maple syrup, one clove of garlic, and a 2" knob of ginger into just a small mixing cup. Blend until smooth, thick, and creamy.

2. Place into a bowl and mix the red and green cabbage thinly sliced, cilantro, carrots, and green onions. Now pour dressing over the mixture of cabbage and toss it to blend.

3. Put the coleslaw in the fridge and cover it before placing inside. Chill for 1 hour.

Note

- For saving time and make this vegan coleslaw even simpler, use a pack of pre-shredded carrots.

- Salt the cabbage so that slaw doesn't get soggy before dressing it to draw out the excess liquid in case of few days in the fridge. It is an additional move, but it is worth the effort.

- Using a spoon to peel the skin off of the ginger knob, cut off the slice of ginger that is to be used for the dressing. In an airtight jar, place the peeled ginger and store that in the freezer. For months, it will remain fresh, and freezing the ginger makes it really easy to grate.

- Keep the leftover coleslaw for 3-5 days in the fridge in an airtight jar.

Nutrition

Kcal 66, fat 2g, Protein 3g, net carbs 11 g

6. Lemon Garlic Oven Roasted Asparagus

Cook time: 12 mins, Servings: 4 servings, Difficulty: easy

Ingredients

- Asparagus (about 25-30 stalks) 1 lb

- Olive oil1 tbsp.

- Dried thyme1/4 tsp

- Onion granules 1/4 tsp

- Lemon zest1 tsp

- Himalayan sea salt and pepper(to taste)

- Lemon slices 4-5

- Cloves of garlic(minced)

- Olive oil 1 tsp

- Fresh lemon juice 1 tbsp.

- Vegan parmesan cheese 1-2 tbsp.

Instructions

1. The oven is preheated to 425 ° first.

2. Wash and dry the asparagus quite well. Prep the asparagus: Wash and dry the asparagus quite well. Either bend the asparagus in half part and let it snap normally, or cut off the base of the stalk by 1 to 1 1/2 inches.

3. Spread the asparagus spears on a tray lined with parchment. Drizzle the asparagus with over 1 tbsp. Olive oil and stir to coat each slice. Sprinkle uniformly over the asparagus following ingredients: thyme, onion granules, pepper, sea salt, and lemon zest, and toss it for one more time. Use lemon slices to top and bake for 8 minutes.

4. Mince the cloves of garlic and place them into the bowl. Take one teaspoon of olive oil and blend it together. Take off the tray from the oven after cooking the asparagus for 8 minutes and spread the minced garlic uniformly over the tray. Take the tray back in the oven and bake for an additional 3-4 minutes.

5. When the asparagus gets tender and not mushy, remove it from the tray. The color should still be bright green.   Over the asparagus, squeeze the half lemon juice (about 1 tbsp.) and top it with finely grated vegan parmesan cheese.

Note

- For this recipe, use one whole lemon. Next, zest the lemon using a Micro plane. Then slice the lemon in half and set aside one half for the juice, and then cut the other half for garnish.

- 1 /2 tsp of garlic powder can be substituted for the additional step of adding the fresh minced garlic.

- Do not add the fresh garlic too soon, and it will burn and taste very bitter if you're doing it.

- Cut off the woody sides of the asparagus before roasting.

- If lemon juice is added before cooking, instead of roasting, the asparagus can steam into the liquid. It's always going to taste fine, but not going to get those tasty little crispy edges.

- Be cautious not to overcook the asparagus; continue to check it. If it's not bright green upon picking it up, it's soft and bendy; then it's probably overcooked.

Nutrition

Kcal 67, fat 4g, Protein 2g, net carbs 5 g

6. Paleo broccoli fried rice (whole30, keto)

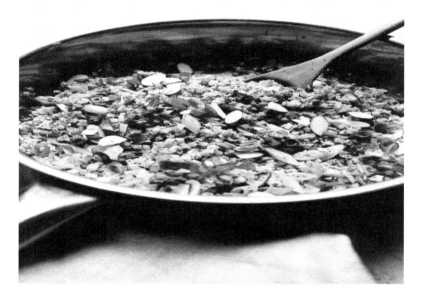

Cook time: 3 mins, Servings: 4, Difficulty: easy

Ingredients

- Two heads riced broccoli 4 cups.
- Ghee/ avocado oil1 tbsp.
- Finely Chopped garlic1 tbsp.
- Coconut aminos1 tbsp.
- Toasted sesame oil1.5 tsp
- Coarse salt(to taste)
- Frozen ginger(grated) ¼ - ½ tsp
- A quarter of one lime juice (more for serving)
- Scallions(chopped)2 bulbs
- Chopped cilantro/ parsley (optional) 4tbsp.
- Sprinkle with sliced almonds (optional)

- Optional pairings:
- Scallops (fresh) 8-10
- Medium-sized shrimp(peeled and uncooked) ½ lb
- Coarse salt¼ tsp
- Black pepper⅛ tsp

Instructions

1. Add one tablespoon of ghee to a well-heated skillet. Sauté the riced broccoli in a pan for 1 min along with finely chopped garlic. In order to season riced broccoli, add coconut amino, toasted sesame oil, and coarse salt. Sauté for an extra 2 mins. Broccoli should be cooked until the color is bright green.

2. Take it off the heat and grate about half a teaspoon of frozen ginger over the rice while the broccoli rice will still be warm. It is then seasoned with some lime juice.

3. Now garnish this with scallions, sliced almonds, and cilantro. Serve on the side with additional lime wedges.

Nutrition

Kcal 87, fat 5g, Protein 2g, net carbs 7 g

7. Roasted Vegetable Tofu Tacos

Cook time: 70 minutes, Servings: 10 tofu servings, Difficulty: capable

Ingredients

Roasted Vegetables

- Medium cauliflower 1
- Sliced cremini mushrooms ½ lb
- Bell peppers medium (sliced) 2
- Chili powder 1 tsp
- Cumin 1 tsp
- Onion powder 1 tsp
- Powder of garlic 1 tsp

- Smoked paprika 1 tsp
- Salt ¼ tsp
- Black pepper ¼ tsp

Crumbled Tofu

- Vegetable broth/ water ¼ cup (to sauté)
- Firm tofu (pressed) 1 package
- Red onion medium (diced) 1
- Cloves of garlic (minced) 3
- Tomato paste 1 tbsp.
- Worcestershire sauce 1 tbsp.
- Chili powder 1 tbsp.
- Paprika 1 tbsp.
- Cumin 1 tbsp.
- Salt ¼ tsp
- Black pepper ¼ tsp

Taco Ingredients

- Spinach tortillas 8
- Head butter lettuce 1
- Avocado (sliced/large) 1
- Hot sauce

Instructions

1. To extract excess liquid, squeeze the tofu into a press for about 30 minutes. One can also cover the tofu block in a dish towel if there is no available press and put a heavy container on top of it.
2. Roasted Vegetables
3. Firstly get the oven preheated to 400 degrees.

4. Upon two big silicone-lined trays, organize the cauliflower florets, sliced mushrooms, and then sliced bell peppers.

5. Sprinkle the vegetables with chili powder, garlic powder, onion powder, smoked paprika, cumin, salt, and black pepper and toss generously to coat. Now bake it for duration of 30 minutes or till all is soft and the tips of the cauliflower florets are of light brown color.

Crumbled Tofu

1. Place the pan over medium heat; while the vegetables get roasted, sauté the chopped red onion in the vegetable broth until it gets soft and translucent in appearance. If the pan looks too dry, add more liquid.

2. The minced garlic, tomato paste, and vegan Worcestershire sauce should be added next. Place it on the heat for an additional 2 minutes while stirring.

3. Move everything else to one side of tray and crumble the block of pressed tofu around the other side of the saucepan with your hands. Sprinkle over the tofu with chili powder, smoked paprika, pepper, cumin, and salt. Stir the tofu to coat with seasonings and then mix together all in the pan. Reduce the heat down to medium-low and cook the mixture for at least about 10 minutes, frequently stirring until thoroughly warmed.

4. The roasted vegetables must be prepared at the same time as the mixture of tofu is ready. Low-carb wraps, roasted vegetables, lettuce, butter, a scoop of tofu crumbles, avocado slices, and a splash of hot sauce make the tacos.

Note

- Try using a firm or extra-firm tofu for the best texture.

- To have a dry or form texture, press and drain the tofu before transferring to the pan and thus have a dry, firm texture.

- Try to stop overcrowding the sheet pans. The vegetables will only steam instead of roasting if the pan is too crowded.

- Keep the leftover filling for 4-5 days in an airtight jar in the fridge or freeze it for a later meal.

Nutrition

Kcal 118, fat 5g, Protein 7g, net carbs 13 g

8. Keto Roasted Radishes

Cook time: 30 minutes, Servings: 6 servings, Difficulty: easy

Ingredients

- Radishes 20-25
- Vegetable broth 1/2 cup
- Medium cloves of garlic(minced) 3
- Dried rosemary1/2 tsp
- onion powder1/2 tsp
- Dried oregano1/4 tsp
- Salt1/4 tsp
- Black pepper1/4 tsp
- Fresh rosemary one sprig (optional)

Instructions

1. Firstly the oven is preheated to 400°.

2. By cutting off the leaves, greens, and roots, prepare the radishes. Well, rinse them. Then slice every radish in half. Quarter them so that they cook quickly if the radishes are any larger than a quarter.

3. Now pour the vegetable broth and add minced garlic, rosemary, oregano, salt, black pepper, and onion powder into a standard size baking dish. To mix the seasonings, whisk it well.

4. Transfer all the radishes to a baking dish, spoon the broth over each one of the radishes to coat, and afterward cover and bake for about 30-35 minutes (check whether the radishes are on the small side for 25 minutes) or until the radishes are soft, stirring midway through.

5. Garnish prior to serving with new rosemary. Place the leftovers for about 4-5 days in an airtight jar in the refrigerator.

Note

- Should choose those radishes that seem to be similar in size so that they are evenly roasted.
- Should roast the raw vegetables in a casserole dish so they remain hydrated since they are not coated in oil while roasting.
- Place the leftovers for 4-5 days in an airtight jar in the fridge.

Nutrition

Kcal 25, fat 1g, Protein 1g, net carbs 1 g

9. Vegan Garlic Aioli

Cook time: 5 mins, Servings: 8 servings, Difficulty: easy

Ingredients

- A cup of original veganaise 3/4 cup
- Garlic cloves medium (minced) 3
- Lemon juice about 2.5 tbsp.
- Himalayan pink sea salt 1/4 tsp
- Black pepper 1/4 tsp

Instructions

1. In a bowl, add all the ingredients and use a whisk to mix. Now cover and refrigerate prior to serving for 30 minutes.
2. Note
3. Press the palm strongly on top of the lemon before cutting the lemon and roll it back and forth to loosen up the juice.
4. If possible, use fresh garlic to add more flavor than dried seasonings.
5. Place the leftover aioli for 5-7 days in an airtight jar in the fridge.

6. Need not freeze the remaining vegan garlic aioli because it does not have the same consistency as the vegan mayo separates.

Nutrition

Kcal 138, fat 14g, Protein 1g, net carbs 2 g

Chapter 8: Desserts recipes

1. Paleo (low carb) cinnamon sugar donuts

Cook time: 15 mins, Servings: 12mini donuts, Difficulty: easy

Ingredients

- Eggs (room temp) 2 large
- Almond milk (unsweetened) 1/4 cup
- Apple cider vinegar 1/4 tsp
- Vanilla extract 1tsp
- Melted ghee 2tbsp
- Granulated monk fruit sweetener /swerve 1/4 cup.
- Blanched almond flour(fine) 1 cup
- Coconut flour ½ tbsp.
- Xanthan gum ¼ tsp
- Ground cinnamon 1tsp
- Baking powder one half tsp
- Sodium bicarbonate(Baking soda) half tsp
- Sea salt 1/8

Topping choices:

For the Cinnamon Sugar Coating:

- Granulated monk fruit /granulated erythritol /swerve 1/4 cup
- Ground cinnamon 1tsp
- Melted ghee / butter 1 1/2 tablespoons
- For the Chocolate Glaze:
- Dark chocolate (sugarless) melted 2 ounces.
- Coconut oil 1tsp
- Powdered monk fruit sweetener 1tsp

Instructions

1. Whisk the eggs, almond milk, vanilla, apple cider vinegar, melted ghee, melted ghee & monk fruit sweetener altogether in a large mixing bowl, until smooth and mixed.

2. Combine the almond and coconut flour, baking powder, xanthan gum, cinnamon, some sodium bicarbonate, and salt in an individual medium dish. Now mix the remaining ingredients to the wet components slowly and mix until they are just blended.

3. Uniformly shift batter into a greased mini donut pan of 12 cavity silicone.

4. Now bake to a preheated 350F oven for 12-15 minutes till we have the golden brown color there.

5. Put off the pan from oven & carefully remove it until it is cool enough to touch the donuts.

For the cinnamon coating:

1. Stir the granulated sweetener and cinnamon together in a shallow dish while the donuts are baking.

2. Melt ghee in a smaller sized heat-safe cup.

3. Now take over each cooling donut and dip lightly in melted ghee, after which roll into the cinnamon/sweetener's coating.

4. Redo this with the rest of the donuts.

For the chocolate glaze:

1. To a small heat-safe mug, add the finely chopped chocolate and coconut oil & melt them in the microwave. Add the sweetener until mixed.

2. Now the cooled donuts are dipped into the chocolate and put in the refrigerator till the chocolate coating is set.

Nutrition

Kcal 86, fat 8g, Protein 2g, net carbs 2 g

2. Keto Peanut Butter Balls

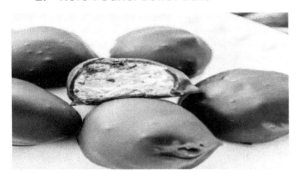

Cook time: 20 mins, Serving: 18, Difficulty: easy

Ingredients

- Salted peanuts chopped 1 cup.

- Peanut butter 1 cup

- Powdered sweetener such as swerve

- Sugar-free chocolate chips 8 oz.

Instructions

1. Mix the sliced peanuts, peanut butter, and the sweetener altogether. Distribute the 18-piece dough and shape it into balls. Place them on a baking sheet lined with wax paper. Refrigerate it until cold.

2. In the microwave or on top of the double boiler, melt the chips of chocolate chips. Let the chocolate chips stay in the microwave, stirring every other 30 seconds unless they are 75% melted. And then just stir until the rest of it melts.

3. Now each ball of peanut butter is dipped into the chocolate, and bring it back on the wax paper. Until the chocolate sets, put it in the fridge.

Nutrition

Kcal 194, fat 17g, Protein 7g, net carbs 7 g

3. Keto Sopapilla Cheesecake Bars

Cook time: 50mins, Servings: 16 bars, Difficulty: capable

Ingredients

Dough Ingredients:

- Mozzarella shredded/ cubed 8 oz.
- Cream cheese 2 oz.
- Egg 1
- Almond flour 1/3 cup
- Coconut flour 1/3 cup
- Joy filled eats sweetener 2 tbsp.
- Vanilla 1 tsp
- Baking powder 1 tsp

Cheesecake Filling Ingredients:

- Cream cheese 14 oz.
- Eggs 2
- Joy filled eats sweetener ½ cups.
- Vanilla 1 tsp
- Cinnamon Topping:
- Joy-Filled Eats Sweetener 2 tbsp.
- Cinnamon 1 tbsp.
- Butter (melted) 2 tbsp.

Instructions

1. First, we pre-set the oven and heat it to 350.
2. Place cheese in a bowl that is microwave-safe. Place for one minute in a microwave. Yeah, stir. Microwave it for 30-second. Stir again. All the cheese ought to be melted at this stage. Microwave it for about   30 more seconds before uniform and gloopy (it should be like cheese fondue in appearance at this

point). Add in the food processor, the remainder of the dough ingredients and the cheese. Mix until a uniform hue by using a dough blade. Wet your hands when it is uniform in color and put half of it into an 8x8 baking dish. On the piece of parchment paper, press the other remaining half into an 8x8 rectangle.

3. Now add the cream cheese, vanilla, eggs, and then sweetener to the food processor to start making the cheesecake filling. Mix into the food processor/ electric blender until smooth.

4. Now the cheesecake batter is poured on top of the bottom part of the dough. Place over the other piece of dough gently on top and peel the parchment paper off. Sprinkle the cinnamon and sweetener on the top of it and glaze with the melted butter.

5. Bake till it is puffed up and golden brown in color, for about 50-60 minutes. Brush over the top with the help of a pastry brush over the last 20 minutes of baking if the butter collects in the middle.

Nutrition

Kcal 190, fat 16g, Protein 6g, net carbs 4 g

4. Best Keto Brownies

Cook Time: 20 mins, Servings: 16 brownies, Difficulty: easy

Ingredients

- 1/2 cup
- Three quarter cup
- 3/4 cup
- 1/2 tsp baking powder
- One tablespoon instant coffee optional
- 10 tablespoons butter (or 1/2 cup + 2 Tblsp)
- 2 oz dark chocolate
- Three eggs at room temperature
- ½ teaspoon optional

Instructions

1. Set the oven, preheated to 350 degrees. Now place an 8x8 inch or 8x9 pan with the layer of aluminum foil, parchment paper, or grease it with butter.

2. Whisk and blend the almond flour, cocoa powder, baking powder together along with erythritol and instant coffee in a mixing cup of medium size. Better make sure that whisk out almost all the clumps of erythritol.

3. Melt the butter and chocolate in a broad microwave-safe bowl and let it stay for about 30 seconds - 1 minute or till it melts. Whisk in the vanilla and eggs and then gradually stir in the dry ingredients until mixed. Be careful not to mix the batter over for a long time, or it's going to get cakey.

4. Move the batter to a baking dish and bake for about 18-20 minutes or until the inserted toothpick comes out wet. Cool in the refrigerator for at least about 30 minutes to 2 hours, and then slice into 16 smaller pieces.

Nutrition

Kcal 116, fat 11g, Protein 2g, net carbs 3 g

5. White Chocolate Peanut Butter Blondies

Cook time: 25 mins, Servings: 16 blondies, Difficulty: easy

Ingredients

- Peanut butter ½ cup
- Butter (Softened) 4 tbsp.
- Eggs 2
- Vanilla 1 tsp
- Raw cocoa butter (Melted) 3 tbsp.
- Almond flour ¼ cup
- Coconut flour 1 tbsp.
- Joy filled eats sweetener ½ cups.

82

- Cup of raw cocoa (chopped) ¼ cup

Instructions

1. At first, the oven is heated to 350. Then cooking spray is sprayed on the base of a 9 x 9 baking dish.

2. Blend the very first five ingredients via an electric mixer until smooth. Flour, sweetener, and chopped cocoa butter are added. Arrange on a baking dish. Bake for about 25 minutes till the middle no more jiggles, and the edges are golden brown in color.

3. Cool properly, and then chill for at least 2-3 hours in the refrigerator before cutting.

4. Note

5. Use the blend of xylitol, erythritol, and stevia, which is twice as sweet as sugar.

6. Very concentrated sweeteners in this recipe do not work.

Nutrition

Kcal 103, fat 9g, Protein 3g, net carbs 2 g

6. Keto Blueberry Lemon Cheesecake Bars

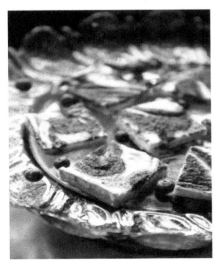

Cook time: 20 mins, Servings: 12, Difficulty: easy

Ingredients

Almond Flour Crust

- butter 8tbsp
- almond flour 1 1/4 cup
- swerve sweetener 2tbsp
- Low Carb Blueberry Sauce
- blueberries 1 1/2 cup
- water 1/4 cup
- confectioners swerve sweetener 1/3 cup
- Lemon Cheesecake Layer
- block cream cheese 1/8 ounce
- egg yolk 1
- confectioners swerve 1/3 cup
- lemon juice 1tbsp
- lemon zest(packed) 1tsp
- vanilla extract 1tsp

Coconut Crumble Topping

- Butter 2tbsp
- Almond flour 1/4 cup
- Coconut flakes(unsweetened) 1/4 cup
- Swerve sweetener 1tbsp

Instructions

1. To start preparing the Blueberry Sauce, add blueberries, sweetener, and water to swerve. Enable the mixture to boil for approximately 10-15 minutes before it becomes thick. Place aside.

2. An oven is preheated for the crust at 350 degrees.

3. Through a foil or parchment paper, cover an 8x8 sheet.

4. Combine in a mixing bowl the melted butter, almond flour and swerve and drop into the pan lined with foil.

5. Prebake crust for about 7 minutes. It must not be firm, only starting to get brown around the edges slightly.

6. Remove and allow the crust to cool. While it is hot, DO NOT add the cheesecake layer.

For the Lemon Cheesecake Layer:

1. Blend in the cream cheese, the yolk of egg, sweetener, and lemon juice, zest, and remove until fluffy and smooth by using an electric mixer.

2. Spread the layer of cheesecake uniformly over the crust.

For the Blueberry Layer:

1. Over through the cheesecake mixture, pour the made low carb blueberry sauce.

For the Crumble:

1. In a blender/ food processor, mix butter, almond flour, unsweetened coconut, and sweetener and also process till it represents a mixture-like crumb.

2. Spread over the blueberry layer over it.

3. Bake until the top is lightly brown in color for 18-20 minutes.

4. Enable the bars to cool before slicing fully.

Note

- To get nice clean slices, put the bars in the freezer for 15 minutes prior to slicing.

Nutrition Facts

Kcal 256, fat 19.9g, Protein 4g, net carbs 6.6 g

7. Espresso chocolate cheesecake bars

Cook time: 35 mins, Servings: 16, Difficulty: medium

Ingredients

For the chocolate crust:

- Butter(melted) 7tbsp
- Blanched almond flour 2 cups
- Cocoa powder 3tbsp
- Granulated erythritol sweetener 1/3 cup
- For the cheesecake:
- Full fat cream cheese 16 ounces
- Big eggs 2
- Granulated erythritol sweetener 1/2 cup
- Espresso instant powder 2 tbsp
- Vanilla extract 1tsp
- Cocoa powder for dusting.

Instructions

The chocolate crust:

1. Preheat the oven to 350° F.
2. Combine the cocoa powder, melted butter, almond flour, and sweetener in a medium-sized dish and blend nicely.
3. Shift the crust of dough to a 9 x 9 pan.
4. Place the crust to the bottom of the dish.
5. The crust is then baked for 8 minutes.
6. Take it off from the oven and set it aside to cool.

Cheesecake filling:

1. Combine the espresso powder, cream cheese, sweetener, eggs, and vanilla extract in a blender and blend until smooth.
2. The crust is poured over the par-baked crust and spread out uniformly into the pan.

86

3. Bake the cheesecake bars at 350° F for 25 minutes, or until set.

4. Remove from the oven and cool.

5. Dust with optional cocoa powder if using.

6. Chill for at least 1 hour, and cut into four rows of squares to serve.

7. Store in an air-tight container in the refrigerator for up to 5 days, or freeze for up to 3 months.

Nutrition

Kcal 232, fat 21g, Protein 6g, net carbs 5 g

8. Pressure Cooker Keto Ricotta Lemon Cheesecake

Cook time: 40 mins, Servings: 6, Difficulty: medium

Ingredients

- Cream Cheese 8 oz.
- Truvia 1/4 cup
- Ricotta cheese 1/3 cup
- Zest of lemon 1
- Lemon Juice 1/4 cup
- Lemon Extract 1/2
- Eggs 2

For topping

- Sour cream 2tbsp
- Truvia 1tsp

Instructions

1. Use a stand mixer; blend all ingredients, excluding the eggs, till a smooth mixture with no granules is left.
2. Now taste it to verify the sweet according to liking.
3. Put the two eggs, deduce the speed and blend gently until the eggs are added. Over-beating can result in a cracked crust at this point.
4. Place into a 6-inch spring-form oiled pan and wrap in foil or a silicone lid.
5. Put two water cups and a trivet in the inner liner of the Instant Pot. Position the foil-covered bowl on the trivet.
6. Cook about 30 minutes at high pressure, and allow it to release the pressure gradually.
7. Combine and spread the sour cream and Truvia on the warm cake.

8. Now refrigerate it for about 6-8 hours.

Oven Instructions

- Prepare the ingredients for the cheesecake as described in the Instant Pot directions.

- Create a water bath and put the pan with the ingredients for the cheesecake inside.

- Bake for about 35 minutes at 375F.

Nutrition

Kcal 181, fat 16g, Protein 5g, net carbs 2 g

9. Keto Ginger Cookie Recipe

Cook time: 15 mins, Servings: 18 cookies, Difficulty: easy

Ingredients

- Cream Together
- Butter/ coconut oil (softened) 4 tbsp.
- Agave nectar 2 tbsp.
- Eggs 1
- Water 2tbsp
- Add Dry Ingredients
- Superfine Almond Flour 2.5 cup
- Truvia/sugar 1/3 cup
- Ground ginger 2tsp
- Ground Cinnamon 1 tsp
- Ground Nutmeg 0.5 tsp
- Baking Soda 1 tsp
- Kosher Salt 0.25 tsp

Instructions

1. First, get the oven preheated to 350F.

2. Now line the baking pan with parchment paper and set it aside.

3. Mix butter, agave nectar, egg, and water altogether.

4. Transfer all the dried ingredients to this mixture and blend well at a reduced speed.

5. Now roll into 2 tsp balls and place them on a baking tray which is lined with parchment paper. They just don't spread too far, but they leave a little gap between them.

6. Bake till the tops become lightly brown in color for about 12-15 minutes.

7. Keep in an air-tight jar when cooled. For, like, an hour before you eat them all, cookies would be around.

Nutrition

Kcal 122, fat 10g, Protein 3g, net carbs 5 g

10. Cream Cheese Pound Cake | Keto Pound Cake

Cook time: 40, Servings: 8, Difficulty: easy

Ingredients

- Cream Cheese(room temperature) 4 ounces

- Softened butter 4tbsp

- Swerve / Truvia 0.5 cup

- Almond Extract 1tsp

- Eggs 4

- Sour cream 1/4 cup

- Superfine Almond Flour 2 cups

- Baking Powder 2tsp

Instructions

1. First, the oven gets preheated to 350 degrees. Grease a 6-cup pan and set it aside. By using a paddle attachment on the

blender, beat the butter, cream cheese, and swerve together in a broad mixer bowl until light and fluffy and well blended.

2. Now pour the almond extract and blend thoroughly.

3. The eggs and sour cream are added and then blend well.

4. Mix all the dry ingredients until they are mixed well. Blend the mixture until light and fluffy.

5. Drop the batter into greased pan. Bake it for about 40 minutes until it comes clean with a toothpick inserted into the bottom.

6. Cut slices and freeze individual slices for a quick sweet tooth remedy,

7. Try beating the batter nicely.

8. Just use a Bundt pan for six cups, not the big 10-12 cup pan

Nutrition

Kcal 304, fat 27g, Protein 9g, net carbs 7 g

Chapter 9: Keto candy and confections

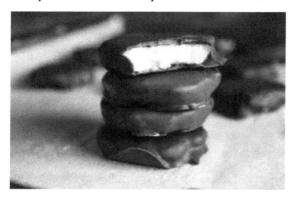

1. Keto Peppermint Patties

Cook time: 5 mins, Servings: 12 patties, Difficulty: easy

Ingredients

- Coconut oil (softened slightly) 0.5 cup
- Coconut cream 2 tbsp.
- Swerve sweetener powdered 0.5 cup
- Peppermint oil /extract 1 - 2 tsp
- Sugar-free chopped dark chocolate 3 ounces.
- Cocoa 0.5 cup

Instructions

1. Put the coconut oil and the coconut cream with each other in a medium bowl until smooth. Whisk together the powdered sweetener tin and 1 tsp of the peppermint extract. If needed, taste and add extra extract.

2. Cover the baking sheet with either parchment or waxed sheets. Dollop onto the paper a heaping tablespoon of the mixture and spread out to a circle of 1 1/2 inches. Repeat the step with the remaining available mixture and freeze for around 2 hours, until solid.

3. Melt together the chocolate and cacao butter in a heatproof bowl positioned over a pan of merely simmering water. Stir until smooth.

4. Drop into the molten chocolate and toss to cover while dealing with one frozen patty at that same time. Remove the extra chocolate with a fork and tap gently on the side of the bowl to remove it.

5. Now put either on a lined tray with parchment paper or wax and leave to set. Repeat the same with the remaining patties.

Nutrition

Kcal 126, fat 13.6g, Protein 0.4g, net carbs 2.9 g

2. Sugar-Free Marshmallows

Cook time: 5 mins, Servings: 10 servings (about 20 marshmallows), Difficulty: easy

Ingredients

- Water 1 cup
- Grass-fed gelatin 2.5 tbsp.
- Swerve sweetener(powdered) 2/3 cup
- Bocha sweet/ xylitol/ allulose 2/3 cup
- Cream of tartar 1/8 tsp
- Pinch salt
- Peppermint extract / vanilla extract 1 tsp

Instructions

1. Line an 8x8 pan with waxed/ parchment paper and grease the paper gently.

2. Mount the stand mixer with the whisk attachment. Through the cup, pour half of the water and brush with the gelatin. When mixing the syrup, let it stand.

3. Mix the rest of the water, the sweeteners, the tartar cream, and the salt in a pot over medium heat. Bring the sweeteners to a boil while stirring.

4. Try bringing the mixture to 237F to 240F temperature using a candy thermometer or an instant-read thermometer. Please remove it from the heat.

5. Set the stand mixer to low and add on the hot syrup slowly down the side of the bowl. Add the extract until all of the syrup is blended in. Adjust the stand mixer to medium-high and beat till the mixture is white, thickened, and lukewarm. It can take 5 to 15 minutes for this.

6. Working fast, pour the blend into the prepared pan dish and smooth the top. Enable 4 to 6 hours until the top is no tackier to the touch.

7. Flip and cut to the appropriate size on a cutting board. If needed, dust with powdered sweetener. Let sit in the air for a day to dry a little, then store in a ziplock container.

Nutrition

Kcal 14, fat 8 g, protein 1.5g, net carbs 0.1 g

3. Keto Sugar-Free Marzipan

Cook time: 30 mins, Servings: 16 servings. Difficulty: easy

Ingredients

- Almond flour 1.5 cups
- Swerve sweetener (Powdered) 1 cup.
- Large egg 1
- Almond extract 2 tsp
- Rosewater 0.5 tsp

Instructions

1. In a food processor, position the blanched almonds and process them until finely ground. Jump to step 2 if the almond meal is used.

2. To mix, introduce the powdered sweetener and pulse. Further, add the egg white, almond extract, and rose water (if consuming) and operate the processor on high until the mixture has become a paste and starts to form a ball.

3. A little extra almond meal is added if the mixture is just too wet. A bit of water, like one teaspoon, is added at a time if the dough seems dry. In texture, it should imitate cookie dough or pastry.

4. Shape into two logs and cover them in plastic wrap tightly. They are usually used for cookies, cake, or candies.

5. Keep the dough tightly packed for a week in the fridge or up to two months in the freezer.

Nutrition

Kcal 65, fat 5.3g, Protein 2.5g, net carbs 2.3 g

4. Keto Rocky Road Fudge

Cook time: 30 mins, Servings: 20 servings, Difficulty: easy

Ingredients

- Homemade marshmallows (sugar-free)3/4
- Heavy whipping cream 1.5 cups
- Bocha sweet 6 tbsp
- Swerve sweetener(powdered) 6 tbsp
- Butter 1/4 cup
- Unsweetened chocolate(chopped) 6 ounces
- Vanilla extract 1 tsp
- Pecan halves 1.5 cups

Instructions

1. Form the marshmallows as per the instructions, but use vanilla extract for replacing the peppermint extract. For drying out properly, these would need to be made a day in advance. Break the marshmallows into 1/2 inch bits and put them on a

sheet of cookie lined with parchment paper. Place it in the refrigerator for a minimum of 3 hours.

2. Now line a 9x13 pan with parchment paper.

3. Whisk together both the cream and sweeteners in a broad pan over medium flame. Boil it and then turn the heat down and bring to a simmer for about 30 minutes. Watch closely that it only simmers but does not begin to boil. Small bubbles should be around the edges the entire time.

4. The butter, chopped chocolate, and vanilla extract are added and are withdrawn from the heat before. Sit for 5 minutes until the chocolate and butter have fully melted, then mix until smooth and fluffy.

5. Now the marshmallows and the pecans are to be frozen. Into the prepared pan, distribute the whole mixture evenly. Cool until set, for about three hours, before slicing into squares.

Nutrition Facts

Kcal 155, fat 14.7g, Protein 1.6g, net carbs 2.3 g

5. German Chocolate Truffles

Cook time: 15 mins, Servings: 20 to 24 truffles, Difficulty: easy

Ingredients

- Whipping cream 0.5 cup
- Egg yolks 2
- Swerve sweetener(powdered) 0.5 cup
- Salted butter (sliced into four pieces) 1/4 cup
- Vanilla extract 0.5 tsp
- Unsweetened shredded coconut 3/4 cup
- Pecans (chopped, toasted) 2/3 cup
- Coconut flour 1tsp
- Sugar-free dark chocolate(chopped) 3 ounces
- Cocoa butter / coconut oil 0.5

Instructions

1. First, cover the baking sheet with parchment / waxed paper.

2. Mix the cream, yolk of eggs, sweetener, and butter over a saucepan on medium flame. Cook for approximately 10 minutes, until thickened.

3. Take it off the heat and stir together the vanilla, coconut, and pecans. Sprinkle on the floor with coconut flour and then whisk fast to blend.

4. Let the mixture cool for 10 to 20 minutes, occasionally stirring. Scoop out, tbsp.-sized mounds on the baking sheet when it's still soft but not runny (A small cookie scoop works well). There has to be 20-24 mounds. Freeze it for 1 to 2 hours.

5. Heat up the chocolate and cocoa butter with each other in a heatproof bowl over a pan of gently simmering water till smooth. To extract excess chocolate, dip the refrigerated mounds into the chocolate coating with the help of a fork and then tap the fork tightly against the side of the cup to remove the excess chocolate. Return to waxed paper and leave to set for 10 to 20 minutes.

Nutrition

Kcal 232, fat 22.85g, Protein 2.3g, net carbs 6.49 g

Chapter 10: Keto ice cream recipes and frozen treats

1. No Churn Strawberry Ice Cream

Cook time: 20 mins, Servings: 10 servings, Difficulty: easy

Ingredients

- Strawberries 12 ounces
- Both sweet 1/4 cup
- Fat sour cream 1.5 cups
- Vanilla extract 1tsp
- Heavy cream 1.5 cups
- Swerve sweetener (powdered) 1/3 cup

Instructions

1. Add in a blender/ food processor the strawberries and BochaSweet together. Blend it till almost purified, but some bits are still left.

2. Now whisk the sour cream, vanilla extract, and strawberry mixture together in a mixing bowl until evenly mixed.

3. In yet another big bowl, whip the cream until it maintains rigid peaks with the powdered swerve. Pour the whipped cream gently into the strawberry mixture until there are only a few streaks left.

4. It is moved to an airtight container and freeze for at least 6 hours until stable.

5. Keep it in the refrigerator, so the ice cream can freeze pretty hard. Can introduce a few tablespoons of vodka to the strawberry mixture to offset the frostiness.

Nutrition

Kcal 202, fat 18.6g, Protein 1.7g, net carbs 4.41g

2. Keto Peach Ice Cream

Cook time: 45 mins, Servings: 8 servings, Difficulty: medium

Ingredients

- Ripe peaches (peeled/ sliced) 400 g
- Bocha sweet/ xylitol 1/3 cup
- Lemon juice 1 tbsp
- Heavy whipped cream 1.5 cups
- Unsweetened almond/ hemp milk 0.5 cups
- Swerve sweetener 1/3 cup
- Egg yolks 4
- Salt 1/4 tsp
- Glucomannan powder/xanthan gum 1/2 tsp
- Vodka 2 tbsp
- Vanilla extract 0.5 tsp

Instructions

1. First, put the diced peaches in a bowl and mix with the lemon juice and Bocha Sweet. Wait for 30 minutes to macerate so that juices are released, then mash with a large fork or potato masher. They must be mashed possibly well, but a few tiny bits and pieces are fine.

2. Over an ice bath, position a reasonable bowl and set it aside.

3. Now blend the cream, almond milk, and swerve in a broad saucepan over a medium-low flame. Bring it to a simmer, constantly stirring so that sweetener gets dissolved.

4. Whisk the yolk of eggs with salt in yet another bowl until smooth. Now pour about a half cup of the hot cream into yolks, whisking constantly. After this, slowly pour the mixture of egg yolk back into the saucepan, whisking continually.

5. Keep cooking along with whisking continuously till the mixture on the thermometer reaches 170F or thickens sufficiently to cover a wooden spoon's back. Turn off the heat and pour quickly over the prepared ice bath in the bowl.

6. Let the mashed peach puree cool for 10 minutes, then whisk in. Glucomannan is the whisking medium used. Refrigerate it for duration of 3 hours and up to night-time.

7. Mix in the vanilla extract and vodka and slowly pour into an ice cream maker's canister. Churn, as per instructions of the manufacturer. Then shift it to an airtight container once churned, and freeze for another hour or two until solid enough to scoop.

8. Until fully churned, about 1 1/2 quarts of ice cream are formed from this recipe. And therefore, it could really be split into ten servings.

Nutrition

Kcal 211, fat 18.1g, Protein 2.8g, net carbs 6.5 g

3. Sugar-Free Fudge Pops

Cook time: 5 mins, Servings: 8 popsicles, Difficulty: easy

Ingredients

- Heavy cream 1 cup
- Almond/cashew milk (unsweetened) 1 cup
- Swerve sweetener 1/3 cup
- Cocoa powder (unsweetened) 1/3 cup
- Vanilla extract/ peppermint extract 1tsp
- Xanthan gum 1/4 tsp

Instructions

1. In a saucepan, blend together milk, cream, swerve, and cocoa powder over moderate flame. Boil it and then cook by stirring continuously for one minute.

2. Take off the heat and add on peppermint extract while stirring. To combine, mix with xanthan gum and whisk speedily. Cool it for 10 minutes and then shift into Popsicle molds.

3. Freeze for 1 hour, then press wooden sticks into popsicles and then return back to the freezer (wooden sticks are best to have stayed in the pops when taken out of the molds). Freeze for about five more hours before solid.

4. Hover under clean hot running water for 30 seconds or so to loosen molds.

Nutrition Facts

Kcal 118, fat 11.2g, Protein 1.44g, net carbs 3.1 g

4. Low Carb Cannoli Ice Cream

Cook time: 10 mins, Servings: 8, Difficulty: easy

Ingredients

- Whipped cream heavy 1 cup
- Swerve sweetener(Powdered) 1/4 cup
- Bochasweet 1/4 cup
- Ricotta cheese 3/4 cup
- Cream cheese 3 ounces
- Vanilla extract 1 tsp
- Lily's chocolate chips (sugar-free) 1/3 cup
- Chopped pistachios (optional) 1/4 cup

Instructions

1. Beat the cream with the Swerve Sweetener in a mixing bowl once it has stiff peaks.

2. Add the ricotta, cream cheese, vanilla extract, and BochaSweet inside a food processor or blender. Mix thoroughly and also have the sweetener dissolved.

3. Fold in the whipped cream with the ricotta mixture. Then fold in the chocolate chips gently.

4. Layer in an airtight jar and chill for 6 to 8 hours until solid.

Nutrition

Kcal 242, fat 20.7g, Protein 5.3g, net carbs 6.4 g

5. Keto Strawberry Lemonade Popsicles

Cook time: 10 mins, Servings: 8, Difficulty: easy

Ingredients

- Sliced strawberries 1 1/4 cup
- A cup of coconut cream 1 1/4 cup
- Squeezed juice of lemon 1/3 cup
- Swerve sweetener(Powdered) 1/3 cup

Instructions

1. Blend the ingredients till fluffy and smooth. Taste the sweetener and change it to your liking.

2. Put over 3-ounces each into Popsicle molds. To release any air trapped bubbles, strike the molds loosely on the counter a few times.

3. Set wooden sticks into the popsicles around 2/3 of the way. (The mixture must be thick enough to hold the sticks in place, but first, freeze the popsicles for 1 hour, then bring them into the sticks).

4. Now freeze it for at least 6- 8 hours.

5. Warm some water in a kettle in order to unmold the popsicles and run it for 5 to 10 seconds outside of the mold, which is to be released. Tug the stick gently in order to remove the Popsicle.

Nutrition

Kcal 117, fat 11.3g, Protein 0.05g, net carbs 2.7 g

6. Sweet Keto Pie Crust

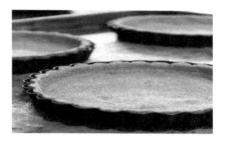

Cook time: 25 mins, Servings: 8, Difficulty: easy

Ingredients

- A cup of almond flour one ¾ cup
- Vanilla/whey protein/ egg white protein powder 1/4 cup
- Erythritol / Swerve(powdered) 1/4 cup
- Egg 1
- Virgin coconut oil/ ghee 2 tbsp.
- Vanilla extract 1 tsp
- Cinnamon 1/2 - 1 tsp
- Pumpkin spice mix 1 tsp
- Food extract (chocolate, almond, etc.,) 1 tsp

Instructions

1. An oven is first preheated to 175 °C/ 350 °F (aided by the fan) or 195 °C/ 380 °F (conventional). All the dry ingredients are blended: the almond flour, whey protein, and powdered Erythritol together.

2. Bring into the coconut oil and egg and process well.

3. Put the dough with a removable bottom in a non-stick pan and press the sides up just to make a "bowl" shape. If required, use a dough roller. Ideally, use a baking sheet as a bottom liner to ensure that the crust does not stick to it.

4. Alternatively, the dough is divided into eight parts and pressed into eight mini tart pans.

5. Position baking paper on top and then weigh the dough down using ceramic baking beans. To avoid the dough from swelling and producing air bubbles, they will be needed, especially if it is a large pie. Locate them inside oven and cook for around 12-15 minutes.

6. Take it out from oven when finished and fill up with your favorite filling (keto lemon flavored curd, chocolate, the whipped cream, creamy textured coconut milk, less-carb custard, some berries, etc.). When not used immediately, let the crust of pie to cool a bit. Keep inside an airtight jar and store at normal temperature for about five days, or freeze for about three months until cooled.

Nutrition

Kcal 181, fat 15.5g, Protein 8.4g, net carbs 2.3 g

7. Low-Carb Cranberry Curd Tarts

Cook time: 30 mins, Serving: 8 tartlets, Difficulty: easy

Ingredients

- A cup of almond flour 2 cups
- Flax meal 4 tbsps.
- Sea salt one pinch
- Butter/ ghee (Unsalted) 2 tbsps.
- Large egg 1
- Low-Carb Cranberry Curd 2 cups
- Heavy whipped cream/coconut cream 1/2 cup

Instructions

1. Get the Low-Carb Cranberry Curd packed. Before using the ad topping, ensure the curd is chilled.

2. Now set the oven to 160 °C/ 320 °F (fan assisted) or 180 °C/ 355 °F to make the pie crust (conventional). Place in a bowl the almond flour, flax meal, and salt and combine to blend. (Note: For a nut-free substitute, one might use an equal amount of ground sunflower seeds.) Add softened butter (ghee/ coconut oil) and eggs.

3. Just use a spoon or hand to blend dense dough is made. Then use a rolling pin, put the dough between two pieces of clinging film, and roll. Shift the dough into a 9-inch tart pan or into eight different 4-inch pans (without the clinging film).

4. Bake for 8 - 10 mins, until nicely browned and crisped.

5. Take the pie crusts out from the oven before introducing the topping and let it cool slightly.

6. Pour the mixture of cranberry curd into each tartlet (approximately 1/4 cup for each tart).

7. Now whisk the cream (coconut cream) in a bowl till bouncy and fluffy. To top each of the tarts, add a dollop of whipped cream by using a spoon.

8. Place it like an hour in the fridge.

9. Sprinkle with cinnamon as a choice and serve.

10. Store for five days in the fridge.

Nutrition

Kcal 366, fat 33g, Protein 8.9g, net carbs 7.2 g

8. Flaky Keto Pie Crust

Cook time: 20 mins, Serving: 8, Difficulty: easy

Ingredients

- Almond flour 2 cups
- Flax meal 4 tbsps.
- Sea salt pinch
- Unsalted butter/ ghee o/ coconut oil 2 tbsps.

- Large egg 1

Instructions

1. First preheat the oven (fan assisted) to 160 °C/ 320 °F or 180 °C/ 355 °F (conventional). Combine the almond flour, flax flour, and a pinch of salt in a dish.

2. Softened (butter/ghee/coconut oil) and egg are poured.

3. Use the spoon or hand to blend until dense dough is formed.

4. Move it to a 9" (23 cm) greased tart pan, eight separate 4" (10 cm) pans, or four specific 5-inch pans. (Suggestion: It's best to use non-stick pie pans with flexible bottoms. Cover the bottom with a sheet of 9-inch (23 cm) round parchment paper if using a big pie pan.)

5. Force the dough down near the bottom and up the sides to make an edge, using either hand or a small roller. It's safer to use baking beans to weigh down the dough and avoid tiny air bubbles from forming while using a large pie crust. Place it into the oven.

6. Depending on the desired brown color, bake for 8 to 12 minutes, rotating the tray halfway to maintain even cooking. Remove the oven tray and put it on a cooling rack. Remove from the pie pans while cooling down. A sharp blade knife can be used to cut gently the pie crusts when needed.

7. Stock for up to 3 days at normal room temperature in a sealed jar, two weeks to refrigerate, or for three months in the freezer.

Nutrition

Kcal 201, fat 18.1g, Protein 6.8g, net carbs 2.3 g

Conclusion

Thus, on a ketogenic diet, you can eat a large range of delicious and healthy meals. These are not just fats and meats. Vegetables are an integral element of the diet. Perfect snacks for a ketogenic diet include meat, olives, nuts, boiled eggs, cheese, & raw vegetables. For intractable seizures, the keto diet offers safe and reasonably balanced treatment. In view of its long experience, however, much remains uncertain about the diet, including its mechanisms of action, the best care, and the broad reach of its applicability. It is possible to limit several of the side effects of beginning a ketogenic diet. Easing into diet & taking supplements with minerals will help. It can be much simpler to adhere to the ketogenic diet by reading food labels, preparing your meals ahead, and carrying your own food while visiting family and friends.

The ketogenic diet usually has special effects on the body and cells, which may have benefits that go well beyond what almost any diet can offer. The combination of carbohydrate restriction and ketone synthesis reduces insulin rates, stimulates autophagy, enhances mitochondrial chemicals' growth and efficiency, reduces inflammation, and burns fat.

CPSIA information can be obtained
at www.ICGtesting.com
Printed in the USA
BVHW060033280221
601200BV00001B/131